Nizar DAOUSSI
Fayez SHTAYEH
Mahbouba FRIH-AYED

Ischemic stroke in the acute phase

Nizar DAOUSSI
Fayez SHTAYEH
Mahbouba FRIH-AYED

Ischemic stroke in the acute phase

Predictive factors and mechanisms of neurological deterioration

ScienciaScripts

Imprint

Any brand names and product names mentioned in this book are subject to trademark, brand or patent protection and are trademarks or registered trademarks of their respective holders. The use of brand names, product names, common names, trade names, product descriptions etc. even without a particular marking in this work is in no way to be construed to mean that such names may be regarded as unrestricted in respect of trademark and brand protection legislation and could thus be used by anyone.

Cover image: www.ingimage.com

This book is a translation from the original published under ISBN 978-620-6-71744-7.

Publisher:
Sciencia Scripts
is a trademark of
Dodo Books Indian Ocean Ltd. and OmniScriptum S.R.L publishing group

120 High Road, East Finchley, London, N2 9ED, United Kingdom
Str. Armeneasca 28/1, office 1, Chisinau MD-2012, Republic of Moldova, Europe
Printed at: see last page
ISBN: 978-620-7-89693-6

CONTENTS

INTRODUCTION

Ischaemic stroke is defined as the sudden and lasting appearance of neurological signs of presumed vascular origin. These signs result from the interruption of blood flow to part of the brain, leading to suffering and necrosis of brain tissue. This condition is one of the main non-traumatic causes of death and disability in adults throughout the world. (1). Its consequences are often devastating for the patient's quality of life, due to the physical dependence and cognitive decline it causes. (2).

Appropriate management of DALYs in the acute phase determines the functional and vital prognosis in the short, medium and long term. This phase represents an important window of opportunity, during which the urgent application of drastic therapeutic measures has a direct impact on patient outcome. Neurological deterioration during this phase is a frequent complication, reported in 2.2% to 37.5% of cases of DALY (3) with a downward trend in recent years according to a recent meta-analysis (4).

Early neurological deterioration (END) is defined as the worsening of clinical neurological signs, measured by the NIHSS score (Appendix), during the acute phase. This extends from a few hours to a few days after the index vascular event (5). DNP is a powerful predictor of poor long-term prognosis (6)Several mechanisms are thought to contribute to the occurrence of this complication, such as the progression of the DVA, loss of collateral circulation, recurrence of the event, cerebral oedema and the spread of thrombi. (7)Numerous factors predictive of DNP have been reported in the literature, including clinical, biological and aetiological parameters. (8).

Identifying these factors in our population will make it possible to target patients at high risk of DNP and develop more effective prevention and treatment strategies, thereby contributing to a significant improvement in the prognosis and recovery of patients suffering from DVA. (9).

The objectives of our study were:

1- Identify factors predictive of DNP following a DALY.

2- Study the mechanisms of this complication

MATERIALS AND METHODS

1. Type of study

This is a cross-sectional, descriptive and analytical study including patients hospitalised at the neurology department of the Fattouma Bourguiba University Hospital in Monastir for DALY over a 5-year period, from 1 January 2018 to 31 December 2022.

2. Study population

We divided our sample into two groups according to whether or not DNP occurred during the acute phase of DALY, after applying the following criteria:

➢ Inclusion criteria :

We included in this study patients who met the following criteria

- Patients hospitalised with a DALY consisting of

- Patients with a minimum follow-up of 7 days

➢ Exclusion criteria :

- Hospital stay of more than 48 hours from onset of symptoms.

- Patients diagnosed with transient ischaemic attack (TIA)

- Missing NIHSS score data at admission and at D7 of follow-up.

3. Definition of early neurological deterioration

We defined NPD as the occurrence of new neurological signs or worsening of pre-existing signs, expressed as an increment (Δ NIHSS) of two points or more in the NIHSS score. In addition, we considered a 7-day window as the temporal criterion for DNP in order to cover the majority of deterioration mechanisms described in the literature.

4. Data collection

The records were searched using the coding of the neurology department of the Fattouma Bourguiba University Hospital in Monastir, using the code "Ischaemic stroke".

We collected socio-demographic, clinical, para-clinical and developmental data from the digital records of hospitalised patients.

The main data collected were :

4.1. Anamnestic data :

We specified patient identification data such as age at onset of DALY, gender and date of hospitalisation, as well as lifestyle habits such as smoking and alcohol consumption.

Personal pathological history, in particular cardiovascular risk factors such as arterial hypertension, diabetes, dyslipidemia, rhythmic and ischaemic heart disease, and previous transient ischaemic attack or DVA were also studied.

We collected chronological data on the vascular event, such as the date and time of onset of various neurological symptoms, with details of the mode of onset, and the time between onset of symptoms and admission to the neurology department.

We compiled information on treatment prior to the onset of the stroke, in particular antiplatelet agents (Aspirin® and Clopidogrel®) and anticoagulants (Sintrom®).

4.2. Clinical examination data

We studied the following clinical parameters:

- Vital signs: heart rate, systolic and diastolic blood pressure.

- NIHSS score on admission, to assess the severity of DALYs and during hospitalisation for up to 7 days.

- Neurological signs: Neurological examination data were carefully collected, in particular the presence of motor or sensory deficits, aphasia with precise type (Broca, Wernické, other), dysarthria, signs of neglect, homonymous lateral hemianopsia, eye deviation, and the presence of a cerebellar syndrome.

4.3. Data from para-clinical examinations

4.3.1. Biological data

The following parameters were collected:

- Blood count: the level of haemoglobin, white blood cells and platelets.

- Inflammation parameters: sedimentation rate and C-reactive protein.

- Glycaemic control data: fasting blood glucose and glycated haemoglobin.

- Renal function and electrolytes: Blood ionogram, uraemia and creatininaemia.

- Lipid profile parameters: total cholesterol, triglycerides, LDL and HDL.

4.3.2. Brain imaging data

We collected the brain imaging data needed to confirm the diagnosis of AVCI and to specify the vascular territory of the ischaemia.

- Cerebral CT: This examination was systematically carried out in all patients in order to rule out differential diagnoses of AVCI and to assess the state of the cerebral parenchyma by looking for the presence of cerebral oedema, haemorrhagic transformation, cortico-subcortical atrophy, leucoariosis, old ischaemic lacunae or sequelae of old cerebral ischaemia. In the case of DNP, this examination is systematically repeated in order to identify the mechanism of the deterioration.

- Cerebral MRI: This is performed in young patients with no vascular risk factors, to help in the etiological investigation and in the search for signs of recent ischaemia using the diffusion sequence.

4.3.3. Data from examinations for aetiological purposes

- Doppler ultrasound of the supra-aortic trunk: This examination is used to detect aetiologies associated with the large trunk, such as atheromatous arterial stenosis and neck vessel dissection.

- ECG, 24-hour rhythm holter and trans-thoracic and trans-oesophageal cardiac echocardiography: This set of aetiological cardiological paraclinical examinations detects potentially emboligenic sources such as the presence of valvular disease, cavitary thrombus or signs of myocardial ischaemia.

- Thrombophilia work-up: blood clotting abnormalities are investigated by measuring Protein S and C, factor V Leiden mutation and anti-thrombin III. A vasculitis work-up is also carried out: This includes testing for inflammatory vasculitides (Lupus, Antiphospholipid Antibody Syndrome, Dry Syndrome, etc.). This work-up is carried out mainly in young patients in the absence of an aetiology in the first-line aetiology work-up.

4.4. Treatment

We studied the different therapeutic options recommended for the aftermath of a stroke. The pharmacological management of DVA is based on thrombolysis in the acute phase and secondary prevention in the long term. Antiplatelet agents are systematically prescribed as soon as the diagnosis of DVA is confirmed. Acetylsalicylic acid (Aspirin®) is the gold standard, prescribed alone or in combination with Clopidogrel (Plavix®). Apart from antiplatelet agents, anticoagulants are indicated in the presence of embolism-inducing heart disease or extracranial carotid dissection. This treatment is based on low molecular weight heparin (LMWH) or unfractionated heparin with per os relay by acenocoumarol (Sintrom®). Statins are routinely used in all patients as part of secondary prevention, with doses adapted to the parameters of the lipid profile, in particular

LDL levels. In the event of cerebral oedema secondary to extensive DALYs, hypertonic solutions (Mannitol®) are recommended.

4.5. Developments

Patient progress was assessed during hospitalisation and subsequently at the outpatient clinic one week after hospitalisation if the length of stay on the ward was less than one week. The NIHSS score was applied as soon as the patient was admitted to hospital and then repeated every day during the patient's stay on the ward.

We adopted as the definition of DNP the loss of two points on the NIHSS score during the first seven days from the date of hospitalisation. In the group of patients meeting the definition of DNP we identified the mechanism responsible for this complication. These mechanisms were classified into 4 main groups, including recurrence of acute phase DVA, haemorrhagic transformation, cerebral oedema and DVA progression. We also studied the occurrence of non-neurological complications such as infection (pneumonia, urinary tract infection), thromboembolic complications (venous thrombosis, pulmonary embolism) and pressure sores during the acute phase of stroke.

5. Statistical analysis :

Statistical analysis was carried out using the Statistical Package For Social Science (SPSS version 22.0). The various variables in the study were tested for normality using the Kolmogorov-Smirnov and Shapiro-Wilk tests. Qualitative variables were summarised by absolute numbers and percentages, while quantitative variables were described by means with standard deviations or medians with interquartile ranges, depending on normality. The Chi-square test (or Fisher's exact test) and the T-test (or Mann-Whitney test) were applied according to the type of variables studied and whether or not the sample was normally distributed. Binary logistic regression was used to identify factors independently associated with the occurrence of DNP. The occurrence of DNP was considered as the dependent variable. The explanatory variables introduced into the multivariate analysis model were those significant at the 5% threshold.

6. Bibliographic research

The bibliographic search was performed mainly on ≪Science Direct≫,≪Springer≫ and the search engines ≪Pubmed≫ and ≪Google Scholar ≫.

The main keywords used were combinations of the following words:

≪Ischemic stroke≫, ≪Early neurologic deterioration≫, ≪pathogenesis≫, ≪Acute≫, ≪prognosis≫, ≪stroke risk factors≫, ≪predictors≫, ≪mechanisms≫, ≪recurrence≫, ≪progression≫ and ≪outcome≫.

Endnote X5 was used to process the bibliographic references.

7. Ethical considerations

Our study was carried out in compliance with ethical considerations. We ensured the confidentiality of patient information by guaranteeing their anonymity throughout the study. Personal and medical data were treated securely and confidentially, in accordance with current regulations. The data extracted from patient files was used exclusively for the purposes of scientific research in this study.

RESULTS

A- Descriptive study

In this study, we included 489 patients hospitalised for a DVA event. These patients were selected after exclusion of 62 patients who did not meet the inclusion criteria or had at least one exclusion criterion (Figure 1). The patients were collected in the neurology department of the Fattouma Bourguiba University Hospital in Monastir over a 5-year period, from 1 January 2018 to 31 December 2022.

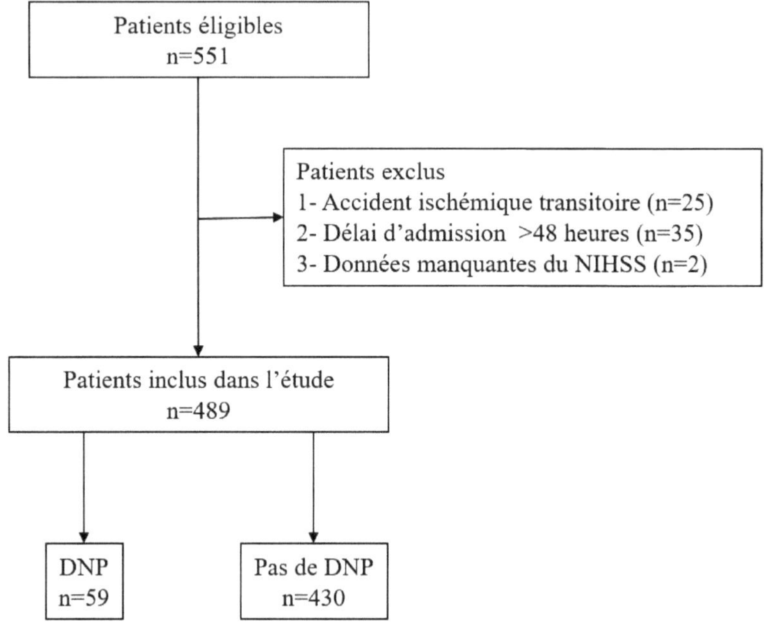

Figure 1Flow chart of patients taking part in the study

I. Socio-demographic characteristics

1. Age

The mean age of our study population was 64.3 years, with a standard deviation of 11.8 and extremes of 24 and 90 years. The peak frequency was between the ages of 60 and 69. The age distribution of the sample also showed that around three-quarters of patients (n=385; 78.7%) were aged between 50 and 79 (Figure 2).

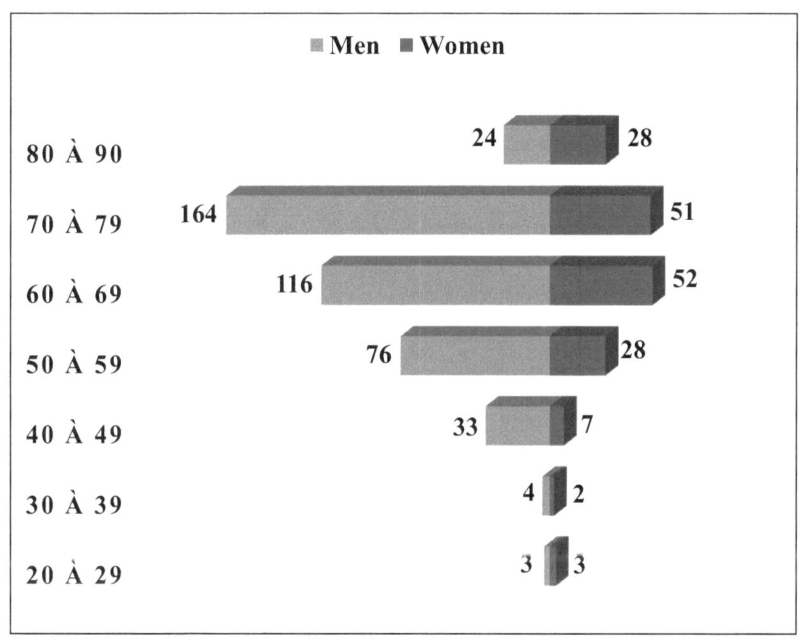

Figure 2Breakdown of patients by age and gender

2. Gender

Sixty-five per cent of patients were male, with a male/female sex ratio of 1.86. We found that males predominated in almost all age groups (Figure 2).

3. Smoking

Active smoking at the time of DALY was reported by 165 patients (33.7%), the majority of whom were male (98.1%).

4. Alcoholism

Consumption of alcoholic beverages was noted in 25 patients (5.1%). These patients were almost all male.

II. Personal medical history

1. High blood pressure

The presence of arterial hypertension among the antecedents was noted in 300 patients (61.3%).

2. Diabetes

Half of our study population (n=244, 49.9%) had diabetes at the time of the DALY, with a predominance of non-insulin-dependent diabetes (77.3%).

3. Dyslipidemia

One hundred and seventeen of our patients (23.9%) were being monitored for dyslipidaemia at the time of hospitalisation for DALY.

4. Cardiovascular diseases

A history of ischaemic heart disease was noted in 67 patients (13.7%). In addition, 67 (13.7%) of our patients were being monitored for a rhythm disorder such as atrial fibrillation, 24 (35.8%) of whom were on anticoagulant therapy.

5. Previous vascular events

The occurrence of a DVA or TIA prior to the index event with a delay of more than one month was noted in 73 (14.9%) and 14 (1.7%) patients respectively.

6. Distribution of vascular risk factors

Figure 3 shows the distribution of the various vascular risk factors. Arterial hypertension (61.3%) is the most common DRF, followed by diabetes (49.9%), smoking (33.7%) and dyslipidemia (23.9%).

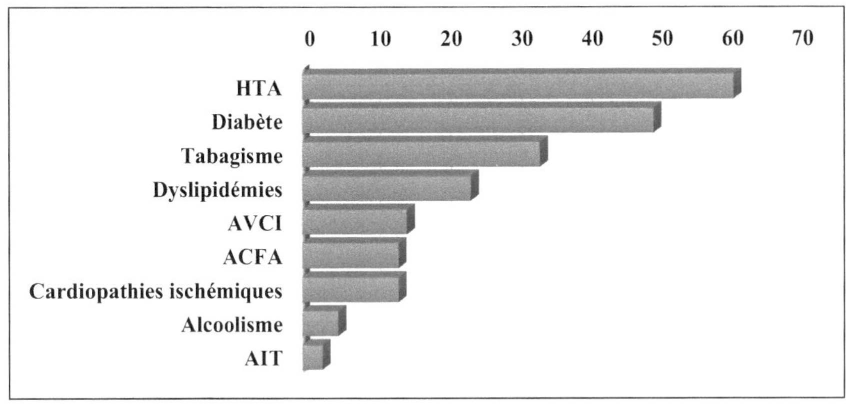

Figure 3Distribution of vascular risk factors

Forty-six of our patients (9.4%) had no vascular risk factors, while two-thirds of the population (65.8%) had at least two (Table I).

Table IDistribution of patients according to the number of vascular DRFs

Number of vascular DRFs	0	1	2	3	>3
Number of employees (n)	46	121	129	110	83
Percentage (%)	9,4	24,7	26,4	22,5	17

III. CLINICAL EXAMINATION Data from the clinical examination

1. NIHSS score

The median NIHSS score on admission was 5 [IIQ=3-9] with extremes of 0 and 25. A study of the severity of the stroke based on the NIHSS score (Fig. 4) showed that 201 patients (41.1%) had a minor stroke (NIHSS between 0 and 4), 250 patients (51.1%) had a moderate stroke (NIHSS between 5 and 15), while 38 patients (7.8%) had a severe stroke (NIHSS>16).

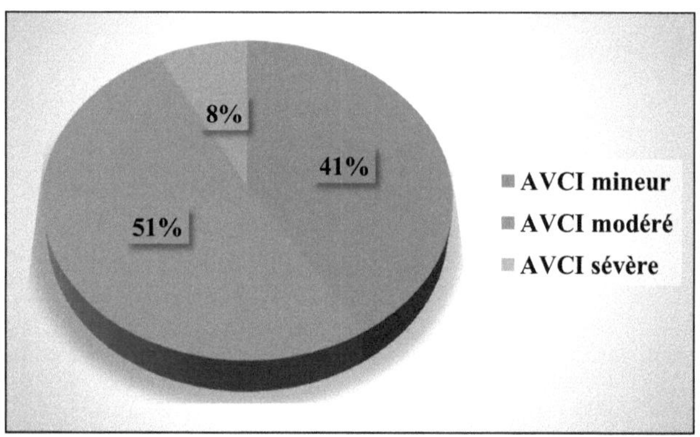

Figure 4Distribution of patients according to severity of DALY

2. GCS score

Fifty-four of our patients (11%) had presented with a disorder of consciousness of varying degrees on admission, with a GCS score of 14 or less.

3. Blood pressure

The mean systolic and diastolic blood pressures at the time of stroke were, respectively, 146 ± 25 mmHg with extremes of 90 and 240 mmHg and 81 ± 13 mmHg with extremes of 50 and 140 mmHg. Three hundred and seventy-three patients (76.2%) had systolic blood pressure greater than or equal to 130 mmHg and/or diastolic blood pressure greater than or equal to 80 mmHg.

4. Heart rate

The mean heart rate in our study population was 80 b/min ±13 b/min with extremes of 50 and 150 b/min.

5. Neurological signs

Analysis of the clinical manifestations of our patients showed that unilateral motor deficit was the most frequent neurological sign. This sign was identified in 329 patients (67.2%). Speech disorders such as dysarthria (paralytic or cerebellar) were noted in 255 patients (52.1%). Hemi-body sensory disorders were identified in 204 patients (41.7%). One hundred and twenty-eight (26.1%) of our patients had aphasia. Of these, 81 patients (16.6%) had Broca's aphasia, 14 patients (2.9%) had Wernické's aphasia and 33 (6.7%) had other types of aphasia. Visual signs such as homonymous lateral hemianopia were noted in 83 (17%) of our patients. Neglect syndrome was reported in 43 patients (8.8%). A cerebellar syndrome was noted in 32 patients (6.5%).

Table IIBreakdown of patients by clinical examination

Clinical characteristics	Number of cases (n)	Percentage (%)
GCS<15	54	11
Motor deficit	329	67,2
Sensory deficit	204	41,7
Aphasia	128	26,1
Broca	81	16,6
Wernické	14	2,9
Other	33	6,7
Dysarthria	255	52,1
Neglect	43	8,8
Hemianopia	83	17
Eye deviation	33	6,7
Cerebellar Sd	32	6,5

IV. Biological test data

Biological data are shown in Table II. The mean haemoglobin level was 13.2 ±1.9 g/dl with a mean platelet count of 232.4 ± 87.6 x 10 /mm[33] .

Hyperleukocytosis and/or elevated CRP were found in 34.7% of patients. A documented bacterial infection, whether pulmonary, urinary or haematological, was noted in 27 patients (5.5%).

Disturbance of the glycaemic balance with elevated fasting blood glucose and/or increased glycated haemoglobin was found in 60.7% of patients. Mean osmolarity was calculated in 233 patients, with a mean of 289 ±9.5. Hyperglycaemic hyperosmolar decompensation was identified in 20/233 patients (8.5%).

The mean LDL cholesterol level in the study population was 2.62 ± 0.95 mmol/l. The majority of our patients (91.7%) had an initial LDL level above the consensus objectives for secondary prevention (LDL > 1.4 mmol/l).

Table IIIResults of biological data

Biological check-up	Average	Standard deviation
Blood glucose (mmol/l)	8,2	3,7
Glycated haemoglobin (%)	7,77	2,36
Creatinine (µmol/l)	84	49
Urea (mmol/l)	6,22	3,17
Sodium (mmol/l)	137	4,1
Potassium (mmol/l)	4,12	0,55
Osmolarity (mmol/l)	289	9,5
CRP (mg/l)	16	32
White blood cells (10 /mm3)^3	8,5	2,8
Haemoglobin (g/dl)	13,2	1,9
Platelets (10^3 /mm3)	232,4	87,6
Cholesterol (mmol/l)	4,46	1,08
Triglycerides (mmol/l)	1,66	0,93
LDL (mmol/l)	2,62	0,95
HDL (mmol/l)	1,07	0,3

V. Brain imaging data

Cerebral CT scans were performed in all subjects in the study. It showed signs of recent DVA in 181 patients (37%) and early signs of ischaemia in 98 patients (20%). This examination was reported as normal or showed old sequelae without signs of recent ischaemia in 210 patients (43%). Only 125 of our patients (25.5%) underwent cerebral MRI.

A study of the arterial territories affected, based on brain imaging data and the clinico-radiological correlation (table III), showed that 347 patients (71%) had presented with a DVA in the carotid territory, 63 patients (12.8%) in the vertebro-basilar territory, 13 patients (2.7%) in junctional territories, while 66 patients (13.5%) had signs of ischaemia in multiple territories.

Table IVDistribution of patients according to DVA vascular territory

Vascular territories	Number of cases (n)	Percentage (%)
Middle cerebral artery :		
Superficial	170	34,5
Deep	68	14
Total	46	9,4
Anterior cerebral artery	13	2,7
Anterior choroidal artery	50	10,3
Posterior cerebral artery	20	4,1
Cerebellar territory	11	2,3
Brain stem	32	6,6
Connecting territories	13	2,7
Multiple territories	66	13,5

VI. Aetiological diagnosis

The aetiological work-up carried out during hospitalisation and follow-up included imaging of the supra-aortic trunks using Doppler ultrasound and/or angioscanner of the neck vessels, and a cardiological work-up to look for embolism-induced heart disease and rare aetiologies. This assessment made it possible to classify the various aetiologies according to the TOAST classification (Figure 5).

In fact, 106 patients (21.7%) had been classified as having DVA of cardioembolic origin, 69 patients (14.1%) had large vessel stenosis in excess of 50% according to the NASCET classification, and 142 patients (29%) had microangiopathic DVA. Other aetiologies, not classified above, such as carotid dissection, were retained in 5 patients (2%). However, the aetiological work-up was inconclusive in a third of cases (n=166; 33.9%), the majority of which were considered to be embolic stroke of undetermined origin (ESUS).

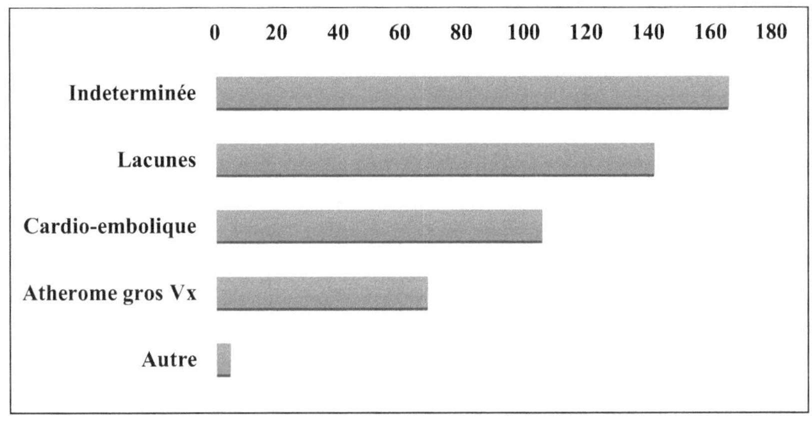

Figure 5Distribution of aetiologies according to the TOAST classification

VII. Treatment

1. Intravenous thrombolysis

Thrombolytic treatment with alteplase (Actilyse®) was administered to patients presenting within the 4.5 hour time window, after checking for any contraindications. In fact, 72 of our patients (14.7%) underwent thrombolysis (Table V).

2. Anti-thrombotic treatments in the acute phase

Antiplatelet agents were prescribed as monotherapy or in combination in 460 patients (94%). Monotherapy with salicylic acid (Aspirin®) or Clopidogrel (Plavix®) was recommended in 314 (64.2%) and 7 patients (1.43%) respectively. The Aspirin-Clopidogrel combination was used in 112 cases (22.9%). Clopidogrel in a loading dose of 300 mg was used in 49 patients (10%). These therapeutic attitudes are in line with the new AHA/ASA recommendations, particularly for minor DALYs.

Anticoagulant treatment with Acenocoumarol (Sintrom®) was prescribed as monotherapy in 13 patients (2.6%) or in combination either with Aspirin® in 26 patients (5.3%) or with Aspirin and Clopidogrel in only one case.

Sixteen patients (3.2%) did not receive anti-thrombotic treatment in the acute phase due to the high risk of bleeding associated with the identification of haemorrhagic transformation and/or the presence of radiological stigmata of amyloid angiopathy.

3. Statins

Statins (Atorvastatin or Rosuvastatin), particularly high-dose statins, were prescribed to the majority of patients (n=479; 98%).

4. Treatment of cerebral oedema

Treatment of cerebral oedema in the acute phase of DVA with hyper-osmotic solutions (Mannitol®) was prescribed in 24 patients (4.9%) with rigorous monitoring of renal function and electrolytes.

Table VTreatments prescribed in the acute phase of DALYs

Treatment administered	Number of employees (n)	Percentage (%)
Intravenous thrombolysis	72	14,7
Anti-thrombotic treatment		
Monotherapy		
Salicylic acid	314	64,2
Clopidogrel	7	1,4
Acenocoumarol	13	2,6
Polytherapy		
Salicylic acid and Clopidogrel	112	22,9
Salicylic acid and Acenocoumarol	26	5,3
Salicylic acid, Clopidogrel and Acenocoumarol	1	0,2
Statins	479	98
Hyperosmolar solution (Mannitol®)	24	4,9

VIII. Frequency of DNP

The occurrence of DNP, as previously defined in our work (ΔNIHSS = initial NIHSS - worsening NIHSS), was observed in 59 patients, i.e. 12.06% of all patients included in the study. The majority of these patients (n=74, 84%) had lost between 2 and 4 points in the NIHSS score (Fig. 6).

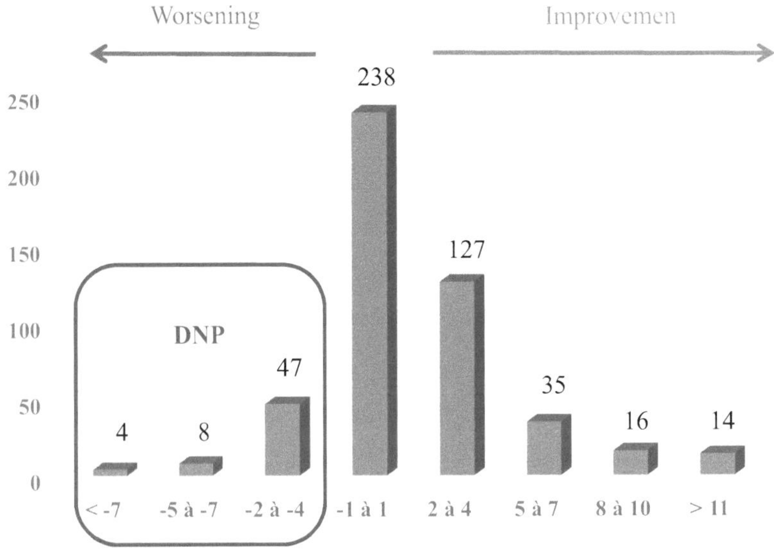

Figure 6Distribution of patients by NIHSS score increment (ΔNIHSS)

IX. Mechanisms of DNP

1. Recurrence of DALY

Recurrence of the DVA during the first week of the index event was diagnosed by the worsening of the initial neurological signs or the appearance of new signs correlated with the identification of new ischaemic lesions on the follow-up cerebral CT scan performed systematically whenever there was a clinical worsening. This situation was recorded in 7/59 patients (11.8%) (Fig. 7).

2. Cerebral oedema

The appearance of cerebral oedema often accompanies extensive strokes, particularly in the carotid territory, and generally occurs within 48 to 72 hours of the stroke. It is confirmed by a follow-up cerebral CT scan.

Of the 59 patients who experienced DNP, six (10.2%) developed cerebral oedema.

3. Haemorrhagic transformation

The worsening of neurological signs was attributed to the occurrence of a haemorrhagic transformation on follow-up imaging in 6/59 patients (10.2%) of those who had a DNP.

4 Progression of the DALY

We considered progression as the mechanism in patients who had a worsening of the initial neurological signs with or without extension of the size of the initial ischaemic lesion and without the appearance of new ischaemic lesions on follow-up imaging. This situation was noted in 40 patients (67%), distributed as follows: a documented infection in 10 patients, decompensation of diabetes in 6 patients and epileptic seizures in 1 case. In the remaining patients with DNP, no cause was identified.

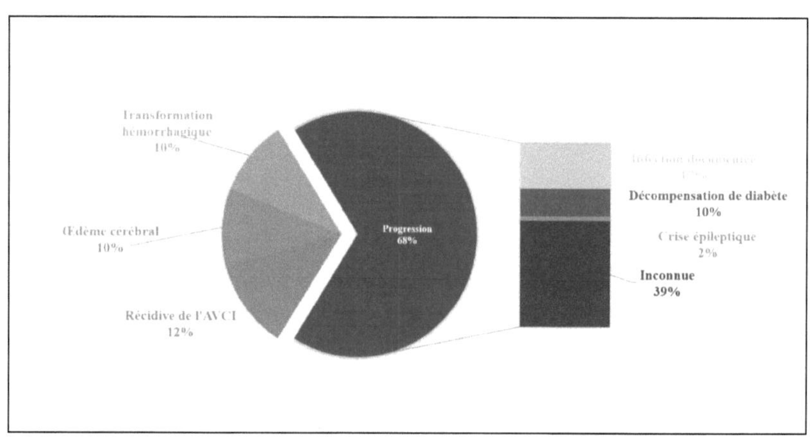

Figure 7Mechanisms of NPD onset

B. Analytical study

I. Univariate analysis

All the variables included in the study and potentially linked to the occurrence of DNP were introduced into a univariate analysis model comparing the group of subjects who had experienced DNP with the rest of the study population.

1. Socio-demographic characteristics

The socio-demographic characteristics studied in our work were age, sex and addictive behaviours at vascular risk (Table VI).

1.1. Age

Patients with DPN had a higher mean age than those without (67.2 years vs 63.9 years). The difference between the mean ages in the two groups was significant (p=0.04). This indicates a correlation between older age and the development of PND after DVA (Table VI).

1.2. Gender

There was no significant difference in the gender distribution of patients (Figure 8). Male patients predominated in both groups (64.2% Vs 71.2%; p=0.29).

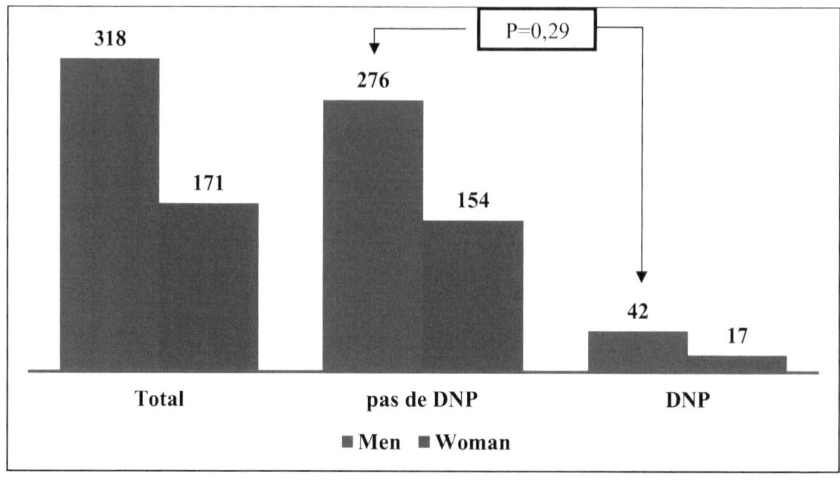

Figure 8Breakdown of NPD by gender

1.3. Smoking

Smoking was higher in patients who had not had DNP, with no significant difference (34.2% Vs 30.5%, p=0.575).

1.4. Alcoholism

The frequency of consumption of alcoholic beverages was comparable in the two groups, with no significant difference (5.1% Vs 5.1%, p=0.992).

Table VISocio-demographic characteristics according to the occurrence of DNP

	Total n=489		No DNP n=430		DNP n=59		p
Age	63,7	(±11,8)	63,9	(±11,7)	67,2	(±11,9)	**0,04**
Men	318	(65%)	276	(64,2%)	42	(71,2%)	0,29
Women	171	(35%)	154	(35,8%)	17	(28,8%)	-
Tobacco	165	(33,7%)	147	(34,2%)	18	(30,5%)	0,575
Alcohol	25	(5,1%)	22	(5,1%)	3	(5,1%)	0,992

2. Personal medical history

The study of the patients' personal histories looked for pathologies that might contribute to an increased cardiovascular risk, and consequently influence the risk of developing PPN after DVA (Table VII).

2.1. History of hypertension

The presence of hypertension in the history was comparable in the two groups (61.2% Vs 62.7%; p=0.819).

2.2. A history of diabetes

The history of diabetes was slightly higher in the group of patients without DNP, with no significant difference (49.3% Vs 54.2%; p=0.477).

2.3. History of dyslipidemia

The frequency of dyslipidaemia in patients' histories was comparable in the two groups (24.2% Vs 22%; p=0.716).

2.4. History of cardiovascular disease

The frequency of coronary heart disease in the patients' history was slightly higher in the group of patients without DNP, with a statistically non-significant difference (14% Vs 11.9%; p=0.662).

On the other hand, the presence of ACFA in the history was slightly higher in the group of patients who had DNP, with no significant difference (15.3% Vs 13.5%; p=0.711).

2.5. History of previous vascular events

The frequency of past DVA in the history was slightly higher in the group of patients who had a DPN, with a non-significant statistical difference (18.6% Vs 14.4%; p=0.393). Similarly, there was no correlation between the presence of past TIAs and the occurrence of PND (p=0.48).

Table VIIDistribution of vascular FDR according to the occurrence of DNP

	Total N=489		No DNP n=430		DNP n=59		p
	(n)	(%)	n	(%)	n	(%)	
Hypertension	300	(61,3%)	263	(61,2%)	37	(62,7%)	0,819
Diabetes	244	(49,9%)	212	(49,3%)	32	(54,2%)	0,477
Dyslipidemia	117	(23,9%)	104	(24,2%)	13	(22%)	0,716
Coronary artery disease	67	(13,7%)	60	(14%)	7	(11,9%)	0,662
ACFA	67	(13,7%)	58	(13,5%)	9	(15,3%)	0,711
AVC	73	(14,9%)	62	(14,4%)	11	(18,6%)	0,393
AIT	14	(2,9%)	13	(3%)	1	(1,7%)	0,480

3. Clinical examination data

Comparing the means of systolic and diastolic blood pressure and heart rate between the two groups, we found no statistically significant difference (Table VII). Similarly, the frequency of altered consciousness (GSC<15) was not statistically different according to the presence or absence of DNP (p=0.123). However, the mean initial NIHSS score in the DNP group was significantly higher than in the rest of the population (9.36±6.7 Vs 6.58±4.6; p=0.002).

Our analysis showed that apart from aphasia (p=0.521), the presence of cortical neurological signs such as neglect syndrome (p=0.018), homonymous lateral hemianopsia (p=0.015) and conjugated head and eye deviation (0.046) was significantly more frequent in the group of patients who had had a DNP (table VIII).

A study of the distribution of patients according to the presence of a motor neurological deficit (p=0.911) or a sensory neurological deficit (p=0.34) did not reveal any statistically significant difference between the two groups. Furthermore, the presence of a cerebellar syndrome was inversely related to the presence of DNP (p=0.023).

Table VIIINeurological clinical signs according to the onset of DNP

	Total n=489		No DNP n=430		DNP n=59		p
Initial NIHSS	6,95	(±5)	6,58	(±4,6)	9,63	(±6,7)	**0,002**
TAS	146	(±25)	145	(±25)	148	(±25)	0,486
TAD	81	(±13)	81	(±11)	80	(±11)	0,294
FC	80	(±13)	79	(±13)	80	(±15)	0,533
GCS<15	54	(11%)	44	(10,2%)	10	(16,9%)	0,123
Motor deficit	329	(67,2%)	288	(67%)	41	(69,5%)	0,911
Sensory deficit	204	(41,7%)	176	(40,9%)	28	(47,5%)	0,340
Aphasia	128	(26,1%)	113	(26,2%)	15	(25,4%)	
Broca	81	(16,6%)	69	(16%)	12	(20,3%)	0,521
Wernické	14	(2,9%)	13	(3%)	1	(1,7%)	
Other	33	(6,7%)	31	(7,2%)	2	(3,4%)	
Dysarthria	255	(52,1%)	220	(51,2%)	35	(59,3%)	0,268
Neglect	43	(8,8%)	33	(7,7%)	10	(16,9%)	**0,018**
Hemianopia	83	(17%)	66	(15,3%)	17	(28,8%)	**0,015**
Eye deviation	33	(6,7%)	25	(5,8%)	8	(13,6%)	**0,046**
Cerebellar Sd	32	(6,5%)	32	(7,4%)	0	(0%)	**0,023**

4. Biological test data

4.1. Blood count

When comparing the mean haemoglobin level in DALY patients with and without DNP, we found no significant difference (8.4 g/dl Vs 9.3 g/dl, p=0.725). Similarly, comparison of the mean platelet count in the two groups showed no significant difference (232.1x10^3 /mm3 Vs 235.1x10^3 /mm3; p=0.817).

However, the mean white blood cell count was higher in the DNP group than in the rest of the study population, with a significant difference (9.34x10^3 /mm3 Vs 8.4x10^3 /mm3; p=0.036).

4.2. Markers of inflammation

Mean CRP levels were significantly higher in patients who had undergone DNP (30 mg/l Vs 20 mg/l; p=0.01).

4.3. Blood glucose levels

We found that the mean fasting plasma glucose on admission was higher in patients with PPN after DALY. This difference was statistically significant (9.22 mmol/l Vs 8.05 mmol/l; p=0.033). However, the comparison of mean glycated haemoglobin levels, reflecting glycaemic control in the months prior to the DALY, did not differ between the two groups (p=0.743).

4.4. Lipid profile

The mean levels of total cholesterol, triglycerides and LDL were comparable in the two groups. However, mean HDL levels were lower in patients with DNP, with a statistically significant difference (0.99±0.27 mmol/l Vs 1.08±0.33 mmol/l; p=0.049).

Table IXCorrelation between biological data and the occurrence of DNP

	Total n=489		No DNP n=430		DNP n=59		p
Blood glucose	8,2	(±3,7)	8,05	(±3,76)	9,22	(±3,11)	**0,033**
HBA1c	7,77	(±2,36)	7,79	(±2,43)	7,67	(±1,82)	0,743
Creatinine	84	(±49)	83	(±40)	96	(±93)	0,102
Urea	6,22	(±3,17)	6,12	(±3,05)	7	(±3,92)	0,128
Na	137	(±4,1)	137	(±4)	137	(±3,9)	0,701
K	4,12	(±0,55)	4,12	(±0,53)	4,09	(±0,67)	0,759
CRP	16	(±32)	14,35	(±25)	32,18	(±62)	**0,01**
GB	8,5	(±2,8)	8,4	(±2,7)	9,3	(±3,2)	**0,036**
Haemoglobin	13,2	(±1,9)	13,3	(±1,9)	13,2	(±1,9)	0,725
Inserts	232,4	(±87,6)	232,1	(±88,6)	235,1	(±80,9)	0,817
Cholesterol	4,46	(±1,08)	4,47	(±1,07)	4,35	(±1,18)	0,451
Triglycerides	1,66	(±0,93)	1,66	(±0,87)	1,69	(±1,33)	0,801
LDL	2,62	(±0,95)	2,62	(±0,94)	2,65	(±1,05)	0,837
HDL	1,07	(±0,3)	1,08	(±0,33)	0,99	(±0,27)	**0,049**

5. Brain imaging data / vascular territories

The superficial territory of the middle cerebral artery (MCA) was affected in 12 patients (20.3%) of those who had DNP compared with 158 patients (36.7%) who did not have this complication (Table X). This difference was statistically significant and inversely related to the occurrence of PPD. On the other hand, the frequency of DALYs in the total territory of the MCA was much higher in patients in the DNP group compared with the rest of the sample (25.4% Vs 7.2%, p=0.013) with a significant difference indicating a strong link between the occurrence of DNP and this vascular topography. Similarly, involvement in the territory of the anterior choroidal artery (AChA) was correlated with the occurrence of DNP (18.6% Vs 9.1%; p=0.03).

Statistical analysis of the remaining vascular territories did not reveal any significant difference in relation to the occurrence of DNP.

Table XCorrelations between vascular territories and the occurrence of DNP

	Total N=489		No DNP n=430		DNP n=59		P
	(n)	(%)	(n)	(%)	(n)	(%)	
ACM							
Superficial	170	34,5	158	36,7	12	20,3	**0,013**
Deep	68	14	60	14	8	13,6	0,913
Total	46	9,4	31	7,2	15	25,4	**<0,001**
ACA	13	2,7	13	3	0	0	0,225
AChA	50	10,3	39	9,1	11	18,6	**0,03**
ACP	20	4,1	19	4,4	1	1,7	0,342
Cerebellum	11	2,3	11	2,6	0	0	0,265
Brain stem	32	6,6	27	6,3	5	8,5	0,612
Junctional	13	2,7	10	2,3	3	5,1	0,267
Multiple	66	13,5	62	14,4	4	6,8	0,116

6. Aetiological diagnosis

We compared the different aetiological classes according to the TOAST classification in terms of the occurrence or non-occurrence of PND in order to identify a possible link between these aetiologies and the occurrence of this complication (Table XI). Our statistical analysis showed that the presence of large vessel atheroma (arterial stenosis of more than 50% of the vessel lumen) was much more frequent in patients presenting with PPN after DVA, with a statistically significant difference (23.7% Vs 13%; p=0.028).

However, we found no significant correlation between the cardioembolic origin of the DALYs and the presence of DNP (20.3% Vs 21.9%; p=0.79). Similarly, we did not find a significant difference between the two groups in the sample with regard to the presence of lacunae (25.4% Vs 29%; p=0.514). DALYs of undetermined aetiology were evenly distributed between the two groups, with a slight increase in their frequency in patients without DNP, with no statistically significant correlation (30.5% VS 34.4%; p=0.522).

Table XICorrelations between the etiologies of DALYs and the occurrence of DPN

	Total n=489		No DNP n=430		DNP n=59		P
	(n)	(%)	(n)	(%)	(n)	(%)	
Cardio-embolic	106	21,7	94	21,9	12	20,3	0,79
Large Vx atheroma	69	14,1	56	13	14	23,7	**0,028**
Gaps	142	29	127	29,5	15	25,4	0,514
Undetermined	166	33,9	148	34,4	18	30,5	0,552
Other	5	2	5	1,1	0	0	-

7. Treatment

The use of intravenous thrombolysis was similar in patients with and without DNP (Table XII). In fact, 13.6% of patients with DNP had undergone thrombolysis compared with 14.9% of thrombolysis in the rest of the study population (p=0.788). Treatment of cerebral oedema with Mannitol® was significantly correlated with the occurrence of DNP (10.2% Vs 4.2%; p=0.046). On the other hand, the different therapeutic modalities prescribed as part of secondary prevention were comparable in the two groups in the sample, with non-significant differences.

Table XIICorrelations between treatments prescribed and the occurrence of DNP

| | Total | | No DNP | | DNP | | p |
| | n=489 | | n=430 | | n=59 | | |
	(n)	(%)	(n)	(%)	(n)	(%)	
Intravenous thrombolysis	72	14,7	64	14,9	8	13,6	0,788
Aspirin	453	89,8	400	93	53	89,8	0,379
Clopidogrel	120	24,5	110	25,6	10	16,9	0,148
Loading dose Clopidogrel	47	9,6	39	9,1	8	13,6	0,273
Preventive LMWH	123	25,2	103	24	20	33,9	0,099
Mannitol	24	4,9	18	4,2	6	10,2	**0,046**
Sintrom	41	8,4	36	8,4	5	8,5	0,979

8. Mechanisms of early neurological deterioration

Statistical analysis identified a strong correlation between early recurrence of the vascular event and the occurrence of DNP. Indeed, the rate of recurrence during the first week of the DALY was 11.9% in the DNP group. In the rest of the sample, this rate did not exceed 1.4% (p<0.001).

Similarly, there was a statistically significant difference in the association between haemorrhagic transformation and the occurrence of DNP. The presence of bleeding on follow-up imaging was noted in 10% of cases of DNP, compared with 1.9% of cases in the rest of the study population (p<0.001).

The occurrence of cerebral oedema in the first few days following DVA was noted in 6/59 patients (10.2%) in the DNP group and only 4.2% in the rest of the patients (p=0.046).

Other plausible mechanisms of PPN were also significantly correlated in the univariate study, such as the presence of a documented intercurrent infection (p<0.001) and hyperosmolar decompensation of diabetes (p=0.027). On the other hand, we did not find any significant association between blood pressure imbalance, impaired renal function, the presence of a bedsore or deep vein thrombosis and the occurrence of DPN.

Table XIIICorrelations between plausible mechanisms and the occurrence of DNP

	Total n=489		No DNP n=430		DNP n=59		p
	(n)	(%)	(n)	(%)	(n)	(%)	
Early recurrence	13	2,7	6	1,4	7	11,9	**<0,001**
Haemorrhagic transformation	14	2,9	8	1,9	6	10,2	**<0,001**
Cerebral oedema	24	4,9	18	4,2	6	10,2	**0,046**
Documented infection	27	5,5	17	4	10	16,9	**<0,001**
Decompensation of diabetes	20	4,1	14	3,2	6	10,2	**0,027**
Epileptic seizures	9	1,8	8	1,9	1	1,7	0,879
Impaired renal function	50	10,2	43	10	7	11,9	0,658
SBT > 160 mmHg	165	33,7	141	32,8	24	40,6	0,312
Eschar	1	0,2	1	0,2	0	0	0,786
Venous thrombosis	2	0,4	1	0,2	1	1,7	0,098

II. Multivariate analysis

1. Analysis of factors associated with NPD

Among the different variables studied in the univariate analysis, fifteen were correlated with the occurrence of PPN during DALY. These variables were entered into a multiple logistic regression model after eliminating confounding factors. In the end, only three variables were independently related to the occurrence of PND (Table XIV).

Table XIVMultivariate logistic regression of factors associated with DNP

Variable	p	Odds Ratio	95% CI
Territory of the anterior choroid	0,002	**5,48**	1,91-15,8
Total forest territory	0,032	**4,11**	1,13-14,9
Atheroma of large vessels	0,012	**3,19**	1,28-7,91

Analysis by multiple logistic regression showed that involvement of the AChA territory (OR=5.84; 95% CI=1.91-15.8) and total MCA (OR=4.11; 95% CI=1.13-14.9) were independent associated factors for the occurrence of PND, with a 4 to 5 fold increase in the risk of this complication. Similarly, DVA of atheromatous origin with significant stenosing plaques (>50%) are independently associated with the occurrence of PTN (OR=3.19; 95% CI=1.28-7.91).

2. Analysis of the mechanisms by which NPD occurs

Several mechanisms of DNP occurrence had shown a statically significant correlation with this complication in the univariate study (Table XIII). Among these mechanisms, those that were significant at the 5% threshold were also introduced into a second binary logistic regression model in order to determine those that were independently involved in the development of DNP (Table XV).

Table XVMultivariate logistic regression of possible mechanisms of DNP

Mechanism studied	p	Odds Ratio	95% CI
Early recurrence of DALY	0,001	**23,2**	3,9-136,9
Intercurrent infection	<0,001	**9,9**	2,9-33,8

Our analysis showed that early recurrence of DVA was an independent mechanism for the development of DPN (OR=23.2; 95% CI=3.9-136.9). The occurrence of a documented infection during the acute phase of DVA also represents an independent explanatory mechanism for DNP (OR=9.9; 95% CI=2.9-33.8).

DISCUSSION

A. Key results

In this study we included 489 patients hospitalised for DALY. The mean age was 64 years (24 to 90 years) with a male predominance (sex ratio M/F=1.86). The incidence of PND in our population was 12.06% (59/489 patients).

Univariate analysis showed that there was a link between the occurrence of DNP and advanced age (p=0.04), the severity of neurological signs estimated by the initial NIHSS score (p=0.002), the absence of a cerebellar syndrome (p=0.023) or cortical neurological signs such as neglect syndrome (p=0.018) and homonymous lateral hemianopsia (p=0.015). Similarly, several biological parameters in the acute phase were linked to the occurrence of DNP, such as fasting glycaemia (p=0.033), increased CRP (p=0.01) and WBC levels (p=0.036), and reduced HDL cholesterol levels (p=0.049). Among the different vascular territories, the identification of ischaemia in the superficial (p=0.013) or total (p=0.001) territory of the ACM as well as the territory of the AChA (p=0.03) was correlated with the occurrence of DNP. The identification of large-vessel atheroma (p=0.028) as an aetiology of DVA was statistically associated with the occurrence of PND.

Our study also described the various plausible mechanisms that could explain the occurrence of DNP. Among these mechanisms, early recurrence (p<0.001), haemorrhagic transformation (p<0.001), cerebral oedema (p=0.046), the presence of a documented infection (p<0.001) and hyperosmolar decompensation of diabetes (p=0.027) were statistically linked to the occurrence of DNP.

Multivariate analysis showed that ischaemia in the AChA territory (OR=5.48; 95% CI=1.91-15.8), or in the total ACM territory (OR=4.11; 95% CI=1.13-14.9) as well as identification of large vessel atheroma (OR=3.19; 95% CI=1.28-7.91) were independent factors associated with PND. Similarly, this analysis concluded that early recurrence of DVA (OR=23.2; 95% CI=3.9-136) and identification of intercurrent infection (OR=9.9; 95% CI=2.9-33) were independent mechanisms of PND.

B. Discussion of the methodology

I. Type of study

This is a retrospective descriptive and analytical study of patients treated intra-hospital for DALY in the neurology department of the Fattouma Bourguiba University Hospital in Monastir, over a 5-year period from 1^{ér} January 2018 to 31 December 2022. This study enabled us to determine the frequency of occurrence of PPN following a DVA as well as the factors associated with this complication. We also identified and analysed the different mechanisms of PND.

II. Choice of population

Our study targeted patients hospitalised in a department specialising in the management of DALYs in order to obtain as much anamnestic, clinical, para-clinical and evolutionary data as possible in relation to this pathology. We used the NIHSS score as a means of measuring neurological worsening. However, the application of this score often poses a problem of reproducibility between the different people who can apply it, such as nurses, emergency physicians and neurologists. (10). This shortcoming was taken into account in our population by selecting patients whose diagnosis and follow-up were carried out by neurologists with ongoing training in the application of the NIHSS score provided by the department's senior neurologists. In addition, systematic daily use of the NHISS score in everyday practice enabled us to detect subtle changes in patients' neurological state and to identify cases of DNP, among other things.

III. Strengths and limitations of our study.

The subject of our study is a frequent and dreaded complication in daily practice that can condition the prognosis of DALYs. This subject is still topical because of the disparity of results concerning its risk factors and exact mechanisms, as well as the existence of imperfections in current preventive measures. In addition, the sample size of our population enabled us to carry out a suitable statistical analysis using multivariate analysis.

However, our study is subject to bias, mainly due to its retrospective nature. An information bias resulting from missing data or imprecise quality in some of the information collected was noted. In fact, our work did not take into account the study of premedication prior to the DVA, which could have a considerable impact on the occurrence of DNP. Furthermore, the analysis of DNP in our study did not take into account the subgroups according to intravenous thrombolysis, which could interfere with the evolution of patients following a stroke. Similarly, the analysis of the radiological data was limited to the precision of the vascular territory without studying the size of the ischaemic lesions, given that the majority of patients are diagnosed by cerebral CT scan, which does not provide sufficient information when the stroke is less than 24 hours old, which is the case for most of our patients. Finally, the mono-centric nature of our study also represents a limiting factor, restricting the extrapolation of our results to other centres that do not systematically hospitalise DALYs in the acute phase.

C. Discussion of the results

I. Frequency of early neurological deterioration

The incidence of DNP in our study was 12%. We defined DNP as the loss of two points in the NIHSS score during the first 7 days following hospitalisation. This definition is not standardised in the literature. Previous studies have applied variable criteria for the clinical assessment of deterioration and the time window of DNP. Still based on the NIHSS score, some authors have defined NPD by a decrement of 4 points or more from this score (11, 12) thus limiting measurement bias. Other authors (13) have adapted a definition based on the NIHSS score items by defining DNP using several criteria at the same time, such as an overall decrement of 2 points or a single point on certain items such as disturbed consciousness (1a, 1b and 1c) or motor deficit (5a, 5b, 6a or 6b).

Siegler et al (14) compared the different cut-off points of the NIHSS score in the definition of DNP. They showed that the 2-point cut-off was the most sensitive in terms of poor functional prognosis and in-hospital mortality. The definition we applied was the most commonly used in the literature (5, 15, 16)It ensures the inclusion of as many cases of DNP as possible, thus covering all the factors and mechanisms associated with this complication.

The frequency of DNP in our population was similar to studies of the same methodology, particularly those adopting the same definition of DNP. In fact, in a multicentre retrospective study (17)which adopted the same definition of DNP as the one we used, involving 29,446 patients, the frequency of this complication was 14.6%. Concerning the authors who adapted the definition of PPD as a worsening of ≥ 4 points of the NIHSS score during the first 72 hours after the onset of the DVA, Chen et al. (18) reported a DNP frequency of 17.9% in a prospective study among 268 patients included in the study. Another retrospective study on a sample of 104 patients concluded that 19.2% of their population had presented with DNP (19). Defining DNP by a single point increment in items 1a, 1b or 1c (level of consciousness), or items 5a, 5b, 6a or 6b (motor deficit) of the NIHSS score occurring in the first 3 weeks after the index event, Kim et al. reported a frequency of DNP in the order of 11% in a large prospective study of 14828 consecutive patients with a DVA.

Table XVI summarises the most recent publications that have looked at the frequency of occurrence of DPN after DALY.

Table XVIFrequency of DNP in the literature

Author	Year	Methodology From the study	Increment NIHSS	Window time	Workforce (n)	Frequency of the DNP
Xu et al (15)	2023	Retrospective	2 points	7 days	442	10%
Liu et al (20)	2022	Retrospective	2 points	7 days	79	40,5%
Yinglin et al (21)	2023	Retrospective	2 points	7 days	241	24,1%
Qiulong et al (22)	2022	Retrospective	2 pt or 1 pt item5	7 days	447	30,8%
Zhang et al (23)	2022	Foresight	2 points	7 days	418	17%
Yue et al (24)	2022	Foresight	2 points	7 days	1330	11,95%
Wang et al (25)	2022	Retrospective	2 points	7 days	375	43,7%
Han et al (26)	2023	Retrospective	1 point	72 hours	267	14,2%
Bao et al (27)	2022	Foresight	2 points	72 hours	732	33%
Nam et al (28)	2023	Foresight	2 pt or 1 pt item5	72 hours	1018	14,4%
Li et al (29)	2023	Foresight	2 points	72 hours	455	10,3%
Jang et al (30)	2023	Foresight	1 pt item5/item1	21 days	492	20,7%
Our study	**2024**	**Retrospective**	**2 points**	**7 days**	**489**	**12,06%**

II. Factors associated with DNP

1. Socio-demographic factors

1.1. Age

In our study, the age of patients with DNP was significantly higher than the rest of the population (67.2 years vs 63.9 years; p=0.04). This relationship was not confirmed in the multivariate analysis. Our results were similar to several studies (31) showing that the age of patients can interfere with DNP without being considered as an independent or main factor. Indeed, a study of 732 subjects aged over 65 years showed that more than a third of this age group had DNP (27).

1.2 Gender

There was no significant difference in the gender distribution of patients. In fact, males predominated in both groups (64.2% Vs 71.2%; p=0.29). Our results are in line with those of a retrospective study of a prospective register of 4060 patients, 54.8% of whom were men (32). No significant difference was found (p=0.408). In contrast, another prospective multicentre study (33) involving 2,641 patients, 40.9% of whom were women, reported that the incidence of NPD was significantly higher in female patients (p=0.002).

1.3. Tobacco

In our study, active smoking was not a factor associated with DNP (p=0.575). In line with our results, several studies have demonstrated that this factor is not necessarily significantly associated with the occurrence of DNP during DALY. In addition, two large prospective multicentre studies with a rate of DNP close to our own (14.1%) reported that smoking was not significantly associated with DNP (5, 34). In contrast, Kim et al. found that active smoking was associated with DNP in univariate analysis without being an independent predictor of END (35).

1.4. Alcohol

Our analysis showed no significant association between the frequency of consumption of alcoholic beverages and the occurrence of DNP (p=0.992). Numerous studies have reached similar conclusions to ours. In addition, Liu et al (11) reported a similar frequency of alcohol consumption between patients in the DNP group and the rest of their population (17.7% vs. 17.3%; p=0.977).

Similarly, another study (36) comparing two groups of patients (with or without DNP) showed no significant correlation between alcohol consumption and the occurrence of DNP, with a value of p=0.8.

2. Anamnestic factors

2.1. Hypertension

In our study, there was no significant association between a history of hypertension and the development of PPD (p = 0.819).

This result is consistent with that of a study (8) of 101 patients showing no significant association between arterial hypertension and DPN (p=0.80). In contrast, a large retrospective study (11) involving 9650 patients, concluded that hypertension was significantly associated with DNP (p < 0.001).

Similarly, Yan et al. (36) showed in a prospective study of 341 patients that a history of arterial hypertension was significantly associated with the onset of DPN, particularly in the case of elevated systolic blood pressure. According to the authors, this relationship is mediated by oxidative stress.

2.2. Diabetes

Our statistical analysis did not identify a significant association between the presence of diabetes and the occurrence of DNP 1 (p=0.477). This finding is consistent with several studies in the literature which have shown that diabetes does not significantly influence the risk of developing DNP (22, 37, 38).

2.3. Dyslipidemia

The frequency of dyslipidaemia in the history of our patients was comparable in the two groups (24.2% Vs 22%, p=0.716). Numerous studies in the literature have reached the same conclusions as ours regarding the history of dyslipidaemia and its relationship with DNP after DVA   (39, 40).

2.4. Cardiovascular history

In our study, the presence of a history of coronary artery disease or atrial fibrillation was not significantly associated with DNP. This result is consistent with several studies that have compared the presence of coronary artery disease (CAD) in patients who had experienced a DALY versus those who did not have a DALY (8, 38, 41).

Similarly, the presence of atrial fibrillation in the patient's history was not associated with DNP (p=0.087) in the study conducted by Nam et al (42). On the other hand, in a retrospective analysis of a large series of over 50,000 patients from the SITS (43)a history of previously known atrial fibrillation at the time of the stroke was associated with the occurrence of PND, although it was not considered to be an independent factor in the multivariate analysis of this study.

2.5. Previous vascular events

Cerebrovascular events prior to the index event, including previous DVA (p=0.39) and TIA (p=0.4) did not influence the risk of PND in our study. This finding is in line with several authors (34, 44) who have shown that these events had no impact on the risk of NPD. However, analysis of the SITS (43) showed a correlation with DALYs (p=0.017) and TIAs (p=0.03) if they occurred in the 3 months preceding the index event.

3. Clinical factors

3.1. Initial clinical severity

The mean initial NIHSS score in our study was significantly associated with DNP (p=0.002) in the univariate analysis. Among other things, patients with a higher NIHSS score were more likely to develop this complication than those with a lower NIHSS score. This result was consistent with the literature. Indeed, Zhang et al. (45) showed that the initial NIHSS score was significantly higher (p<0.001) in patients with DNP, out of a total of 1060 subjects, of whom 193 patients (18.2%) had this complication. Similarly, a retrospective analysis of a larger sample showed that a high initial NIHSS score was independently associated (OR=6.8; 95% CI= 6.8-7.6) with the occurrence of DNP (11). An NIHSS cut-off score >8 was reported to be an independent predictor of a five-fold increased risk of developing PND in patients with DVA (46).

3.2. Consciousness disorders

Altered consciousness (GSC<15) was not statistically associated with DNP (p=0.123) in our study. This result was consistent with that of a prospective study (29) involving 509 patients with 10.3% cases of DNP, which showed that altered consciousness was not associated with this complication (p=0.328). On the other hand, Amer et al. (47) found a significant association between a median GCS of 12 and DNP (p=0.01).

3.3. Blood pressure

In our study, mean systolic and diastolic blood pressures were not correlated with the development of DPN. Similarly, Gong et al. (38) showed that systolic blood pressure was not significantly correlated with the occurrence of DPN (p=0.359). On the other hand, diastolic blood pressure showed a significant association with the occurrence of DNP in this study (p=0.023).

In thrombolysed patients, systolic and diastolic blood pressures were significantly independently related to the occurrence of DNP (OR=2.6; 95% CI=1.5-3.3). In the same study (36)the systolic pressure range between 140 and 149 mmHg had the lowest risk of developing DPN, with a sensitivity of 85.6%. Another recent study (48) compared the different blood pressure targets and showed that the risk of DNP increases in parallel with the increase in blood pressure in the acute phase. The odds ratio increased from 9.3 (95% CI=4.3-20.4) for a SBP target of 160 to 180 mmHg to 16 (95% CI=5.9-42.8) if the SBP exceeded 180 mmHg.

4. Biological factors

4.1. Glycaemic control

In our study, we found that the mean fasting blood glucose level on admission was significantly higher in patients with DPN after DALY (p=0.033). However, the comparison of mean glycated haemoglobin levels, reflecting glycaemic control in the months preceding the DALY, did not differ between the two groups (p=0.743).

This result is in line with the majority of studies in the literature. Lin et al. (26) showed that fasting glycaemia and glycated haemoglobin levels were significantly associated with NPD. In contrast, Lee et al. (49) reported in a study of 178 patients that mean HbA1c was not significantly correlated with DNP in DALY (p=0.196). The glycaemia/HbA1c ratio is an indicator of the stress hyperglycaemia that often accompanies the acute phase of DALYs. This ratio is an independent associated factor of DNP (50).

4.2. Renal function and electrolytes

Analysis of renal function, including creatinine and urea levels as well as electrolytes, showed no link with DNP in our study. This is consistent with the literature (51). However, the uric acid/creatinine ratio was considered to be an independent predictor of DNP (21).

4.3. Biological signs of infection

CRP and white blood cell levels were associated with the development of DPN in our univariate analysis, with p-values of 0.01 and 0.036 respectively. Several other studies (52) have confirmed this statistical relationship. Wang et al. (25) investigated the concomitant study of several indicators of the systemic inflammatory response. This study demonstrated that CRP levels, the neutrophil/lymphocyte ratio and monocyte levels were independent predictors of DNP. The authors of this study particularly highlighted the effect of the systemic inflammatory response index (SIRI), calculated from the neutrophil count multiplied by the monocyte/lymphocyte ratio, as an independent predictor of DNP. Also, the neutrophil/lymphocyte ratio (53) is attracting more interest in the literature as a predictor of DNP.

4.4. Components of the lipid profile

The mean levels of total cholesterol, triglycerides and LDL in our study were comparable in the two groups. However, mean HDL levels were lower in patients with DNP, with a statistically significant difference (p=0.049).

Like our results, Ryu et al (54) demonstrated that low HDL was the only independent predictor of PPD among all lipid parameters. An increase in triglyceride levels was associated with a five-fold increased risk of DNP according to a meta-analysis of 4 prospective studies (55). Another study looking specifically at triglycerides showed that not only was an increase in triglycerides associated with PPD, but also low triglyceride levels. The authors (56) concluded that there was a J-shaped link between triglyceride levels and DNP. New non-traditional lipid markers have recently attracted a great deal of interest in the study of the risk of PPD. The plasma atherogenic index (API) (57) calculated from the logarithmic function of the triglyceride/HDL ratio was an independent predictor of DNP (OR=3.2; 95% CI=1.4-7.1). Similarly, the triglyceride-glucose index (TyG), calculated from the neperian logarithm of the product of triglyceride levels multiplied by blood glucose, played an important role in predicting DNP (16).

4. Radiological factors associated with DNP

4.1. Vascular territories

Among the different radiological data possibly associated with PND, our study showed that ischaemia in the total territory of the MCA (OR=4.11; 95% CI=1.13-14.9) as well as the territory of the AChA (OR=5.48; 95% CI=1.91-15.8) were independently associated with the occurrence of PND. In a study including 38 cases of DALY in the total territory of the AChA (58)the presence of large lesions in the diffusion sequence (DWI>89 cm^3) was the strongest independent predictor of DNP (OR=11; 95% CI=2.31-57.1). The same study showed that the lesion volume cut-off of 89 cm^3 had a specificity of 95.7% and a sensitivity of 85.7% in predicting DNP. The timing of DNP in DVA in the total territory of the MCA was studied in a multicentre review (59) which showed that more than two thirds of DNP cases occur 48 hours after the onset of the DVA. As a result, the occurrence of cerebral oedema with mass effect seems the most likely mechanism in the case of ischaemia in the total territory of the MCA.

The rate of DNP in the AChA territory is particularly high compared with other vascular territories. This rate can be as high as 60% in anterior choroidal infarcts exceeding 15 mm in size (60). Nicolas Chausson et al. (61) reported a DNP rate of 46% by adopting a stricter definition of DNP with a 4-point increment in the NIHSS score during the first three days of DVA. These last two studies showed that the only factor predictive of progression in this arterial territory was an initial NIHSS score greater than 6. DVAs in the AChA territory (Figure 9) may follow a particular clinical behaviour called "capsular warning syndrome" described long ago by Donnan et al. (62) and defined as a cluster of stereotyped sensory-motor deficit "bursts" occurring over 24 to 48 hours. The impact of capsular warning syndrome on the risk of DNP was studied in a recent publication in Neurology (63) which showed a very high risk of deterioration during the acute phase (OR=7; p<0.001).

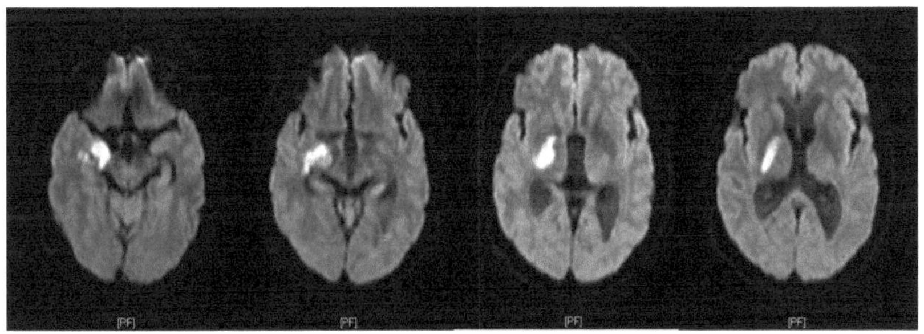

Figure 9Diffusion sequence MRI scan of the brain of one of our patients, aged 54,

The mechanism of DNP in this entity is a matter of debate. The haemodynamic hypothesis has been proposed (64)given that AChA is characterised by a small diameter, less than 1 millimetre on average, emerging from large arterial trunks with high blood flow, such as the internal carotid artery and less frequently the ACM or posterior cerebral artery. Studies based on diffusion tensor mapping (65, 66) have shown that involvement of the pyramidal tract is a factor in DNP in the AChA territory rather than the size of the lesion itself.

With the exception of the total territory of the ACM and that of the AChA, the rest of the territories analysed in our study had no significant association with the occurrence of DNP. Our results are consistent with those of a study (67) involving 1387 patients with a risk of DNP three times higher in the ACM territory compared with the other vascular territories. A recent study analysing subgroups of the prospective Chinese INTERCIS (68) compared the risk of PND between the anterior and posterior cerebral circulation and found no significant difference between these two topographies.

4.2. Other radiological factors

Several other radiological factors, such as the size and nature of thrombi, chronic abnormalities in the FLAIR sequence and the presence of microbleeds, have been shown to have an effect on the risk of DNP. These factors were not analysed in our study because of the difficulties in performing cerebral MRI, which is now the gold standard in the study of DVA.

<u>* Thrombus characteristics</u>

The study of arterial thrombus characteristics (69) showed that thrombus size is a strong predictor of recanalisation failure and consequently of DNP (OR=9.91; 95% CI=3.89-13.87). In addition to the size of the thrombus, its radiological appearance plays a role in the prognosis, particularly in the acute phase of stroke. The calcium nature of the thrombus was identified in only one patient in our series from the DNP group (Figure 10). Indeed, a recent study of the French national thrombectomy registry (70) including a meta-analysis of 135 cases, showed that the calcium nature of the thrombus was correlated with a low rate of recanalisation (TICI 2b) and a poor prognosis at 3 months, with a rate of 28% of patients with mRS of 0 to 2. Another European multicentre study (71) also showed a similar prognosis at 3 months with only 26.5% of patients with mRS 0 to 2 and 55.9% mortality.

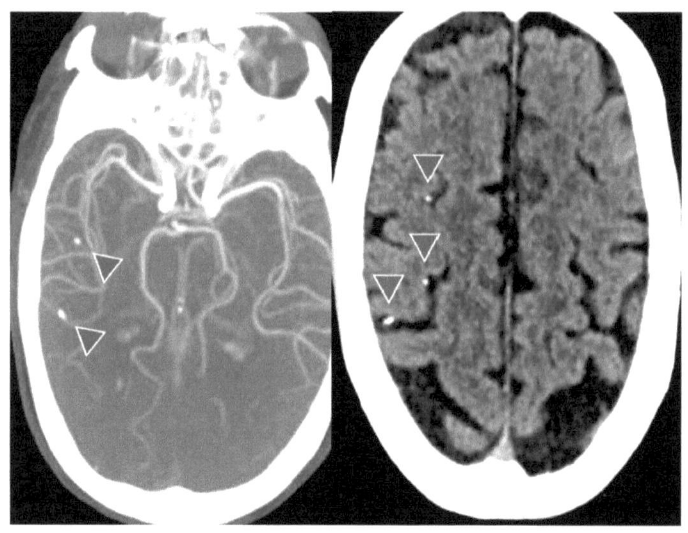

Figure 10Cerebral CT scan in axial sections with and without injection of contrast medium showing spontaneous hyperdensities related to calcium emboli in the arterial pathways (red arrows)

On the other hand, the double-layer clot (Figure 11), which is rich in red blood cells and points to a cardio-embolic origin with a specificity of 97%, was less associated with the occurrence of DNP but rather with a better prognosis following recanalisation procedures. (72, 73) .

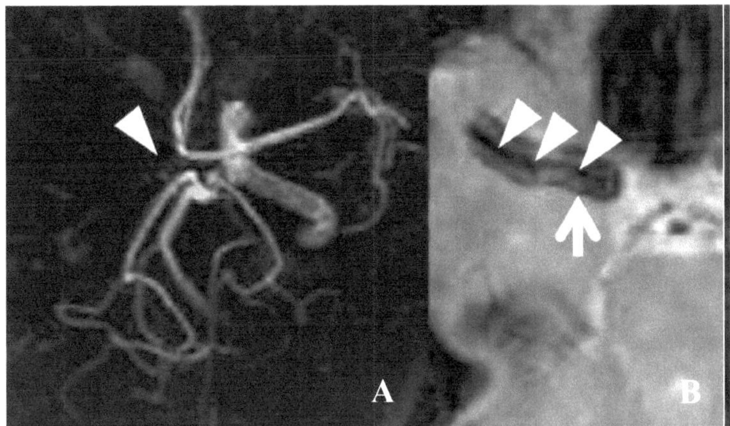

Figure 11(A) Cerebral MRI in 3D-TOF sequences showing carotid-sylvian occlusion (B) T2* gradient echo sequence showing extensive thrombus with double layer appearance (72)

<u>* The presence of microbleeds on the T2* sequence</u>

The term "microbleeds" is used to describe a radiological aspect found on the magnetic susceptibility sequence of cerebral MRI, related to perivascular microhaemorrhages. This aspect often raises a prognostic problem, particularly when making therapeutic decisions during the acute phase of stroke. In one study (74) on 163 patients with microangiopathic DVA, the presence of microbleeds was correlated with the occurrence of PND with an odds ratio of 5.09 (95% CI=1.1-21.7). Aoki et al (75) studied the effect of the presence of microbleeds on 1102 patients treated with dual anti-platelet aggregation therapy, irrespective of aetiology. This study showed no DNP at 14 days or 90 days after DALY. In contrast, another study (76) of thrombolysed patients showed that the presence of more than 5 lobar microbleeds was associated with a poorer prognosis at 3 months (OR=0.57; 95% CI=0.33-0.97) with a three-fold increased risk of symptomatic haemorrhage.

According to the latest recommendations of the European Stroke Organisation (77)the search for microbleeds by cerebral MRI is not recommended, given the considerable delay in treatment. On the other hand, these recommendations contraindicate thrombolysis if the number of microbleeds exceeds ten. A recent review of the literature (78) concluded that, at present, the presence of microbleeds should be interpreted with great caution and stressed the importance of further studies on the risks raised by this radiological factor.

<u>* The presence of white matter abnormalities on the FLAIR sequence</u>

The presence of white matter abnormalities on the FLAIR sequence is a frequent condition found in more than 45% of DALY cases (79). It often reflects the state of the cerebral vascularisation, particularly the collateral supply networks (80). The effect of the presence of these anomalies on the risk of DNP was evaluated in the study by Zhu et al. (81) using the ASPECTS score applied to the extent of white matter lesions. This study analysed patients outside the thrombolysis delay period treated with double anti-platelet aggregation and concluded that the low ASPECTS score, applied to white matter abnormalities, was an independent predictor of DNP (OR=0.39; 95% CI=0.174-0.872). This result was also reported in two other studies (82, 83) which looked at patients with large vessel occlusions. A meta-analysis (79) of 33 prospective studies including a total of 3577 patients showed that white matter abnormalities on the FLAIR sequence constituted a predictive factor for DNP with an overall odds ratio of 1.93 (95% CI=1.3-2.85). A recent study (83) focused on the presence of old ischaemic lacunae rather than vascular leukopathy and showed that the presence of these lacunae is an independent radiological predictor of DFN, particularly in patients with large vessel atheroma.

5. Aetiological factors

In our study, univariate analysis showed that, of the different aetiologies of DALYs according to the TOAST classification, only large-vessel atheroma was associated with the occurrence of PND (p=0.028). This factor was independently associated with PND in multivariate logistic regression (OR=3.19; 95% CI=1.28-7.91). These results are consistent with those of a recent study (8) on patients who lost two NIHSS score points during the first 24 hours with 57% of patients in the DNP group having a DALY related to large vessel atheroma compared with 16.2% in the rest of the population. In this study, a logistic regression model including only the aetiological subtypes showed that cardioembolic and lacunar origin were associated with a much lower risk of developing DNP. Other studies (84, 85) have analysed patients with extracranial atheroma (carotid plaques >50%) and intracranial atheroma (M1 and basilar trunk stenoses) in the same group. These studies always converge towards the same conclusion, which stipulates a very high risk of DNP in these patients, in line with our results.

Like atheroma of the large vessels, the lacunar origin of DVA exposes patients to a risk of DNP with less frequency. A large series published by Siegler et al (67) analysing 947 patients, showed that DNP was identified in only 24.8% of patients whose DVA was of lacunar origin, compared with 46% of DVAs of undetermined origin, 38.5% of patients whose aetiology was large-vessel atheroma and 38.5% of DVAs of cardioembolic origin.

In our study, the incidence of DALYs due to embologenic heart disease was virtually identical in both groups, with and without DNP (20.3% Vs 21.9%). This result is in line with the aforementioned publications (8, 67). In fact, DVA of cardioembolic origin is known for its maximum severity from the outset, leaving little chance of secondary deterioration except in cases of haemorrhagic transformation or malignant DVA (35).

6. Therapeutic factors

In our study, we did not find any statistical association between the different therapeutic modalities considered in the acute phase and the occurrence of DNP with regard to anti-platelet aggregation treatments, anticoagulants, statins and intravenous thrombolysis.

This finding is consistent with the conclusions of a very recent retrospective study (15) adopting the same definition as we used for DNP. This study showed that the use of mono- or dual anti-platelet therapy did not influence the risk of developing DPN. On the other hand, subgroup analysis enabled them to conclude that double anti-aggregation was a risk factor for DNP in cases of minor DVA of undetermined origin. The authors of this study indirectly deduced that DVA of undetermined origin would have an embolic mechanism that responds better to anticoagulant treatment than antiaggregants.

Apart from the absence of any effect on the increased risk of DNP, dual anti-platelet aggregation has shown a preventive effect in relation to the occurrence of this complication in the case of Aspirin-Clopidogrel (86) and Aspirin-Cilostazol (87).

Based on the CHANCE (88) and POINT (89)the current recommendations (90) stipulate the use of double anti-platelet aggregation for 21 days after the occurrence of a minor DALY. This limitation to 21 days is due to the premature termination of the POINT study, given that the significance threshold for bleeding other than intracranial bleeding was exceeded from day 8 to day 90 of the trial. In short, dual anti-platelet aggregation has no effect on the risk of acute phase DNP or on the risk of bleeding during the first week of DALY.

In our study, we were unable to study the effect of statin prescription on DNP because all our patients were systematically treated with statins.

Prescription of statins in the acute phase of stroke has been shown to improve the prognosis and recurrence of stroke (91, 92). It is now universal practice. Jang et al (30) compared the effect of statin doses on the risk of developing DNP. In this observational study, high-dose statins were an independent protective factor against the occurrence of DPN (OR=0.39; 95% CI=0.2-0.75). In contrast, in the randomised clinical trial INSPIRES (93) comparing high-dose Rosuvastatin (20 mg) with low-dose Rosuvastatin (5 mg) for 14 days, the authors found no statistical difference in functional prognosis at 3 months. The ASSORT (94) is a randomised, controlled, multicentre study which compared the early introduction of statins on day one versus a delay of 7 days. This study showed that there was no significant link between the timing of statin introduction and the occurrence of DNP by comparing patients who received statins on the first, second or third day of DALY. The question of the optimal timing for the introduction of statins remains controversial. The SATBRAD (95) designed to answer this question is currently being recruited and will be published in 2026.

III. Mechanisms of DNP

Of the mechanisms suggested in the literature to explain DNP, recurrence of stroke in the acute phase, haemorrhagic transformation, cerebral oedema and progression of stroke are the most studied and best known. (35, 96). In our analysis, we based ourselves on this classification in order to study the plausible mechanisms of DNP, while aligning ourselves with the majority of studies in the literature.

1. Early recurrence

In our study, early recurrence of DVA was noted in 7/59 (11.8%) patients who had experienced DNP. This mechanism was independently linked to DNP (OR=23.2; CI95%=3.9-136). It was selected in the event of worsening of pre-existing neurological signs or the appearance of new symptoms related to the identification of new ischaemic lesions on follow-up imaging performed systematically in the event of any neurological worsening. Our results are consistent with those of Nair et al (97) who demonstrated that the appearance of new ischaemic lesions on brain imaging was a powerful predictor of DNP (OR=10.02; 95% CI=2.81-35.36). A large study (17) involving 29446 patients, with 4299 cases (14.6%) of DNP, showed that recurrence of DVA was the mechanism of DNP in 8.5% of cases. This cohort also analysed recurrence of DVA, as a mechanism of PND, over time and concluded that the frequency of this mechanism increases over time, rising from 3.5% at the first 24 hours to 13.9% at one week from the index event.

A second, more recent study also reported a frequency of early recurrence of DVA as the explanatory mechanism for PND in 163/1717 patients (9.5%) who had experienced this complication. This same study compared patients in whom the mechanism of early recurrence was retained versus patients with DNP related to the progression of the DVA and concluded that cardioembolic origin was statistically associated with recurrence (31.9% Vs 16.6% p<0.001). This finding stems from the fact that cardioembolic strokes generate new strokes in areas other than the initial area. (13).

The study of this DNP mechanism in patients treated with intravenous thrombolysis has demonstrated a very significant impact of this treatment on reducing the risk of recurrence of DVA, which varies between 0.6% and 1.8% in this sub-group of the population (98).

2. Haemorrhagic transformation

Haemorrhagic transformation confirmed by brain imaging was the explanatory mechanism of PND in 6/59 of our patients (10.2%). This was naturally a symptomatic haemorrhagic transformation, since these patients worsened clinically with an increment of at least two points in the NIHSS score according to the definition of DNP that we adopted.

In the Park et al cohort, haemorrhagic transformation was reported in 6.1% of cases. In contrast to the frequency of recurrence of DVA, the frequency of haemorrhagic transformation in this study tended to decrease after the index event. In fact, 10.8% of cases of haemorrhagic transformation occurred during the first 12 hours after the start of the DALY, while only 3% occurred after the third day. (17). A systematic review of the literature including 11 cohorts concerning the etiological mechanisms of DNP in the first 24 hours showed that haemorrhagic transformation was retained as the direct cause of DNP in 3.6% to 7.1% of cases (3). However, the same review showed that this rate rose to 21.4% in patients treated with intravenous thrombolysis. In our study, multivariate analysis of DNP mechanisms did not find an independent link between haemorrhagic transformation and the occurrence of DNP. In fact, several variables could constitute a confounding factor by increasing the risk of haemorrhagic transformation (97) such as increased systolic blood pressure in the acute phase (OR=1.08; CI95%=1.00-1.18) and the presence of a proximal arterial occlusion (OR=3.79; CI95%=1.22-13.99).

3. Cerebral oedema

DNP was associated with the presence of cerebral oedema as the main mechanism in 6/57 patients (10.2%). This mechanism is often evoked when DNP is manifested by headaches and/or a deterioration in the state of consciousness with pupillary or oculomotor abnormalities (99, 100). In the cohort of Nair et al (97)cerebral oedema was identified in 14.7% of DNP cases. In another study (35)whose number of DNP was close to our sample, the frequency of cerebral oedema as a mechanism of DNP was 26.3% (15/57 patients) treated with intravenous thrombolysis. This high frequency is probably due to the high proportion of proximal occlusions that are candidates for recanalisation therapies. In summary, the frequency of cerebral oedema in our population is consistent with that reported in the literature (43, 101, 102) which varies between 6% and 26%. Cerebral imaging confirms this mechanism by demonstrating radiological signs such as deviation of the median line and mass effect on the ventricles in the case of supratentorial stroke, and herniation of the cerebellar tonsils in the case of posterior fossa infarction. Pathophysiologically, cerebral oedema follows a chronological cascade, beginning with cytotoxic oedema which sets in within the first hour and lasts a day on average, characterised by an intact blood-brain barrier with cellular turgidity secondary to a defect in transmembrane ionic transport due to failure of ATP-dependent pumps (103). Vasogenic oedema, secondary to rupture of the blood-brain barrier with extravasation of fluid into the extracellular compartment, occurs 24 to 48 hours after the onset of DALY (104).

4. Progression of the DALY

In our study, DNP was attributed to DVA progression in 40/57 patients (67%). This mechanism is retained after exclusion of the situations described above (recurrence, haemorrhagic transformation and cerebral oedema). The frequency we reported was similar to that described in a large multicentre prospective cohort of 4299 cases of DNP, where progression of the DVA was retained as the causal mechanism in 71.8% of cases (17). In this same study, three quarters of cases of progression occurred within the first 72 hours, with a downward trend to 25% one week after the index event. This mechanism was the most frequent (44%) in the cohort of Nair et al (97) ahead of cerebral oedema and haemorrhagic transformation.

The exact definition of DALY progression as a mechanism of PND is not well established in the literature, which explains its very high frequency with great variability between studies. In fact, this term includes a range of mechanisms, some of which are established and others still hypothetical (96). Several of these mechanisms have not been studied in our cohort due to the lack of adequate radiological investigation methods such as perfusion MRI.

4.1. Collateral circulation failure

The leptomeningeal collateral circulation is a network of emergency vascular anastomoses which is activated immediately after the onset of a stroke. This network supplies hypoperfused areas, leading to a radio-clinical "mismatch" and an extension of the time window for revascularisation therapies. (105). The concept of collateral failure applies essentially to supratentorial AVCI, in the presence of arterial occlusion (106). The failure of this circulation leads to the extension of the necrotic ischaemic lesion at the expense of the penumbral zone. Several studies have confirmed the causal link between poor quality collateral circulation, defined as the presence of collaterals in less than 50% of the infarcted area, and the progression of DVA (107, 108). Inter-individual differences in the quality of the collateral circulation have led to the emergence of the concept of fast and slow "necrosis factors (109)These are based on the speed of progression of the DALY, which is thought to be genetically predefined.

4.2. Progression and nature of the thrombus

In addition to the role played by the failure of the collateral circulation, the extension of the size of the arterial thrombus participates in the progression of the AVCI, and thus in the occurrence of DNP. Indeed, Seners et al reported that PND was independently associated with thrombus elongation (OR=3.96; 95%

CI=1.25-12.53), suggesting a possible mechanism of expansion or re-embolisation of the thrombus in situ (110). This progression would be increased by hyperglycaemia, which would have a pro-thrombotic effect responsible for the increase in thrombus size (111). DNP in this case could result from occlusion of the perforating collateral branches opposite the portions invaded by the thrombus, or from occlusion of the bifurcations more distal to the site of occlusion. On the other hand, the size of the thrombus, estimated by the magnetic susceptibility sequence (T2*), played an important role in explaining the occurrence of DNP. Indeed, He et al. (112) demonstrated that the risk of DNP was 5 times greater if the size of the thrombus exceeded 9.45 millimetres. In addition, a large thrombus was a strong predictor of non-recanalisation following thrombectomy (113). The increasing use of this technique in recent years has highlighted the link between the histological nature of the thrombus and the post-procedural clinical response. Indeed, a recent review of the literature has shown that thrombi rich in red blood cells, frequently associated with cardioembolic origin, are associated with a better rate of recanalisation and require fewer passages during thrombectomy with a better prognosis (114). On the other hand, fibrin-rich thrombi have a higher coefficient of friction, and consequently adhere more to the vascular wall and are more difficult to extract, which exposes them to a high risk of DNP following thrombectomy.

4.3. Epileptic seizures

Epileptic seizures during the acute phase of DALYs or acute symptomatic seizures were noted in 1.8% of cases in our population. These seizures were not correlated with the occurrence of PND (p=0.879). In the literature, they are reported in 1 to 4% of cases of DALY during the first 7 days (115). Certain conditions favour this complication, such as cortical damage, extensive ischaemia and the presence of haemorrhagic transformation (116). Acute symptomatic seizures are often responsible for a transient worsening of the neurological state (Todd's phenomenon). However, prolonged focal seizures and partial malignant states may be responsible for lasting NPD, often explained by the effect of the seizure itself on the infarcted cerebral zone (117).

4.4 Intercurrent infections

Our study showed that 16.9% of patients with DNP had a documented infection, compared with only 4% in the rest of the population. A statistically independent association was found on multivariate analysis (OR=9.9; 95% CI=2.9-33.8). The frequency of occurrence of infections during the acute phase varies in the literature between 5 and 65%, with an average of 30% according to a large meta-analysis of more than 130,000 patients (118). Pulmonary and urinary tract infections were the most frequent, with an approximately equal distribution. In an analysis of the two largest Chinese stroke registries involving more than 700,000 patients (119)the infection rate was 9.6%. The link between infections and the occurrence of PND is an indirect one, involving several explanatory mechanisms (120) such as fever, hypoxia and hypotension. Infection can also affect the evolution of DALYs in several other ways. Prolonged hospitalisation due to infection management delays rehabilitation. In addition, the systemic inflammatory response, through the production of pro-inflammatory cytokines, interleukins and other inflammatory mediators, hinders the recovery process post DALY (121, 122).

The link between infections and PND could be via direct mechanisms of deterioration, as mentioned above, such as recurrent stroke and haemorrhagic transformation. Indeed, Xu et al (119) demonstrated that infection is an independent associated factor for stroke recurrence (OR=1.7; 95% CI=1.65-1.75) and haemorrhagic transformation (OR=3.55; 95% CI=3.34-3.77) during the acute phase.

4.5. Decompensation of diabetes

Fasting blood glucose levels in patients with DNP averaged 9.22 mmol/l, compared with 8.05 mmol/l in the rest of the population, with a statistically significant difference (p=0.033). Similarly, hyperglycaemic hyperosmolar decompensation was more frequent in the DNP group (p=0.027). The majority of studies in the literature agree that hyperglycaemia in the acute phase of DVA has a detrimental effect on the functional prognosis and mortality of DVA. Recently, Yu et al (22) demonstrated that a fasting blood glucose cut-off of 7.15 mmol/l was an independent factor in DNP. The mortality rate increases dramatically to 50% when this threshold exceeds 11.1 mmol/l (123). The exact mechanism explaining the impact of glycaemia on DNP has not been fully elucidated. Endothelial damage, high oxidative stress, lactic acid accumulation and damage to the blood-brain barrier could all contribute to the progression of acute DALYs (22).

4.6 Blood pressure instability

In our study, we did not find any link between systolic or diastolic blood pressure levels and the onset of DNP. However, several studies (124-126) state that blood pressure instability with frequent hypotensive jerks in the first 24 hours increases the risk of DNP (OR=1.2, CI95%=1.01-1.45). This is because falls in blood pressure are responsible for a reduction in cerebral perfusion pressure, which represents the gradient between arterial and venous pressure. Given that the brain tissue located in the penumbra zone is devoid of autoregulatory mechanisms, any drop in arterial pressure will lead to the evolution of oligaemia towards necrosis of the cerebral parenchyma and, consequently, to DNP (127). The deleterious effect of blood pressure has been demonstrated in the case of falls but also in the case of hypertensive peaks with a U-shaped relationship (128). This mechanism currently constitutes a therapeutic target for the management of DNP in the acute phase. Indeed, it has recently been shown that induced hypertension can improve the signs of DNP when started early (129).

CONCLUSION

The sudden onset of neurological deterioration during the acute phase of DALY is a frequent complication. It is a major concern for all those involved in the patient's care, from arrival in the emergency department through to the patient's return home. This complication is important not only because of its consequences in the acute phase, but also because of its definite effect on the functional and vital prognosis of patients in the future. The precise definition of this situation depends essentially on close monitoring of clinical neurological signs using the NIHSS score. It is defined by an increase in this score during the first few days of the DALY. The fight against PPN begins with a good understanding of its probable mechanisms and the associated factors that can prevent or minimise the risk of its occurrence. Although there are a large number of studies on this risk, the factors associated with this complication have not been formally selected because their presence was not uniformly reproduced in the literature. By identifying these factors in our population, it would be possible to target individuals at very high risk of DNP, paving the way for more appropriate and drastic prevention and treatment strategies.

The objectives of our study were:

1- Identify factors predictive of DNP following a DALY.

2- Study the mechanisms of this complication

In order to achieve these objectives, we conducted a retrospective descriptive and analytical study of patients hospitalised at the neurology department of the Fattouma Bourguiba University Hospital in Monastir for a DALY over a 5-year period, from 1 January 2018 to 31 December 2022, including patients meeting the definition of DNP "loss of two points in the NIHSS score during the first 7 days following hospitalisation".

We included patients who had been hospitalised for a DVA and had a minimum follow-up of 7 days. We excluded patients hospitalised after 48 hours of symptom onset and patients with transient ischaemic attack. We excluded files with missing NIHSS score data at admission and at D7 of follow-up.

Our study population consisted of 489 patients. The mean age was 64 years (24 to 90 years) with a male predominance (Sex Ratio M/F=1.86). The incidence of DNP in our population was 12.06% (59/489 patients).

➤ In the univariate analysis, the parameters significantly associated with the occurrence of PPN after DALY were :

- Advanced age

- Severity of neurological signs estimated by the initial NIHSS score

- The presence of neurological signs such as neglect syndrome, homonymous lateral hemianopsia and cerebellar syndrome

- The value of fasting blood glucose

- Increased levels of CRP and white blood cells

- Lower levels of HDL cholesterol

- The presence of ischaemia in the total or superficial territory of the middle cerebral artery and the territory of the anterior choroidal artery.

- Identification of large-vessel atheroma as an aetiology of DVA

➤ The explanatory mechanisms significantly associated with DNP were

- Early recurrence of DALY within the first 7 days of onset of PND

- Haemorrhagic transformation

- Cerebral oedema

- The presence of a documented intercurrent infection

- Hyperosmolar decompensation in diabetes

➤ In multivariate analysis, the independent risk factors for the occurrence of

DNP were :

Ischaemia in the anterior choroidal artery territory (OR=5.48; 95% CI=1.91-15.8), or in the total middle cerebral artery territory (OR=4.11; 95% CI=1.13-14.9) as well as identification of large vessel atheroma (OR=3.19; 95% CI=1.28-7.91) were independent factors associated with PND. Similarly, this analysis concluded that early recurrence of DVA (OR=23.2; 95% CI=3.9-136) and the identification of an intercurrent infection (OR=9.9; 95% CI=2.9-33) were independent mechanisms associated with PND.

The results of our study have led to a number of conclusions:

1- Despite the current multidisciplinary recommendations for the management of acute stroke and the considerable efforts made by all those involved, including emergency physicians, radiologists and vascular neurologists, the incidence of PPN remains high and requires more drastic measures to prevent it.

2- The risk of DNP depends essentially on the clinical condition at the time of the stroke, such as the severity of symptoms, metabolic imbalance, intercurrent infections and vascular territory, as well as aetiology, much more than on the particularities of the terrain in terms of gender and vascular risk factors.

3- Particular attention should be paid to the elderly, who appear to be more vulnerable to this complication.

4- Initial general measures such as strict control of blood sugar and blood pressure and early detection and treatment of infections are a cornerstone in reducing the risk of DNP.

5- In the event of DNP, immediate diagnosis of the causal mechanism by urgent imaging checks and the various biological parameters should be systematically considered in the event of any worsening in order to minimise the serious impact on the patient's subsequent quality of life and future.

REFERENCES

1.	Feigin VL, Stark BA, Johnson CO, Roth GA, Bisignano C, Abady GG, et al. Global, regional, and national burden of stroke and its risk factors, 1990-2019: a systematic analysis for the Global Burden of Disease Study 2019. The Lancet Neurology. 2021;20(10):795-820.

2.	Walter K. What is acute ischemic stroke? Jama. 2022;327(9):885-.

3	Seners P, Turc G, Oppenheim C, Baron J-C. Incidence, causes and predictors of neurological deterioration occurring within 24 h following acute ischaemic stroke: a systematic review with pathophysiological implications. Journal of Neurology, Neurosurgery & Psychiatry. 2014.

4	Martin AJ, Price CI. A systematic review and meta-analysis of molecular biomarkers associated with early neurological deterioration following acute stroke. Cerebrovascular Diseases. 2019;46(5-6):230-41.

5	Liu H, Liu K, Zhang K, Zong C, Yang H, Li Y, et al. Early neurological deterioration in patients with acute ischemic stroke: a prospective multicenter cohort study. Ther Adv Neurol Disord. 2023;16:17562864221147743.

6	Heitsch L, Ibanez L, Carrera C, Binkley MM, Strbian D, Tatlisumak T, et al. Early neurological change after ischemic stroke is associated with 90-day outcome. Stroke. 2021;52(1):132-41.

7.	Kim J-M, Bae J-H, Park K-Y, Lee WJ, Byun JS, Ahn S-W, et al. Incidence and mechanism of early neurological deterioration after endovascular thrombectomy. Journal of neurology. 2019;266:609-15.

8.	Sabir Rashid A, Huang-Link Y, Johnsson M, Wetterhäll S, Gauffin H. Predictors of early neurological deterioration and functional outcome in acute ischemic stroke: the importance of large artery disease, hyperglycemia and inflammatory blood biomarkers. Neuropsychiatr Dis Treat. 2022:1993-2002.

9	Fan J, Li X, Yu X, Liu Z, Jiang Y, Fang Y, et al. Global burden, risk factor analysis, and prediction study of ischemic stroke, 1990-2030. Neurology. 2023;101(2):e137-e50.

10	McLoughlin A, Olive P, Lightbody CE. Reliability of the National Institutes of Health Stroke Scale. British Journal of Neuroscience Nursing. 2022;18(Sup5):S3-S10.

11	Liu P, Liu S, Feng N, Wang Y, Gao Y, Wu J. Association between neurological deterioration and outcomes in patients with stroke. Annals of Translational Medicine. 2020;8(1).

12	Bhole R, Nouer SS, Tolley EA, Turk A, Siddiqui AH, Alexandrov AV, et al. Predictors of early neurologic deterioration (END) following stroke thrombectomy. J Neurointerv Surg. 2023;15(6):584-8.

13	Kim J-T, Lee JS, Kim BJ, Park J-M, Kang K, Lee SJ, et al. Frequency, management, and outcomes of early neurologic deterioration due to stroke progression or recurrence. Journal of Stroke and Cerebrovascular Diseases. 2023;32(2):106940.

14.	Siegler JE, Boehme AK, Kumar AD, Gillette MA, Albright KC, Martin-Schild S. What change in the National Institutes of Health Stroke Scale should define neurologic deterioration in acute ischemic stroke? Journal of Stroke and Cerebrovascular Diseases. 2013;22(5):675-82.

15.	Xu B, Xin X, Ding Y, Xu A, Zhang Y. Effect of Dual-versus Single-Antiplatelet Therapy on Early Neurological Deterioration in Minor Stroke of Undetermined Cause. Acta Neurologica Scandinavica. 2023;2023.

16	Wang J, Tang H, Wang X, Wu J, Gao J, Diao S, et al. Association of triglyceride-glucose index with early neurological deterioration events in patients with acute ischemic stroke. Diabetol Metab Syndr. 2023;15(1):112.

17	Park TH, Lee J-K, Park M-S, Park S-S, Hong K-S, Ryu W-S, et al. Neurologic deterioration in patients with acute ischemic stroke or transient ischemic attack. Neurology.

2020;95(16):e2178-e91.

18   Chen Z, Cao T, Zhong X, Wu Y, Fu W, Fan C, et al. Association between serum netrin-1 levels and early neurological deterioration after acute ischemic stroke. Frontiers in Neurology. 2022;13:953557.

19   Chen N-H, Zhang Y-M, Jiang F-P, Liu S, Zhao H-D, Hou J-K, et al. FLAIR vascular hyperintensity predicts early neurological deterioration in patients with acute ischemic stroke receiving endovascular thrombectomy. Neurological Sciences. 2022;43(6):3747-57.

20   Liu H, Zhang Y, Fan H, Wen C. Risk Factors and Functional Outcomes with Early Neurological Deterioration after Mechanical Thrombectomy for Acute Large Vessel Occlusion Stroke. Journal of Neurological Surgery Part B: Skull Base. 2022;84(02):183-91.

21   Liu Y, Wang H, Xu R, He L, Wu K, Xu Y, et al. Serum uric acid to serum creatinine ratio predicts neurological deterioration in branch atheromatous disease. Frontiers in Neurology. 2023;14:1098141.

22.   Yu Q, Mao X, Fu Z, Luo S, Huang Q, Chen Q, et al. Fasting blood glucose as a predictor of progressive infarction in men with acute ischemic stroke. Journal of International Medical Research. 2022;50(10):03000605221132416.

23   Zhang K, Liu H, Zong C, Yang H, Wang A, Wang Y, et al. Lesion Location Predicts Early Neurological Deterioration in Single Subcortical Infarction. Current Neurovascular Research. 2022;19(5):487-94.

24   Liu Y, Zhao J, Li F, Sun H, Sun Y, Yang F, et al. Predictive value of hemoglobin level on early neurological outcomes in acute ischemic stroke. Neurological Research. 2022;44(8):684-91.

25   Wang J, Zhang X, Tian J, Li H, Tang H, Yang C. Predictive values of systemic inflammatory responses index in early neurological deterioration in patients with acute ischemic stroke. J Integr Neurosci. 2022;21(3):94.

26.   Han L, Hou Z, Ma M, Ding D, Wang D, Fang Q. Impact of glycosylated hemoglobin on early neurological deterioration in acute mild ischemic stroke patients treated with intravenous thrombolysis. Front Aging Neurosci. 2023;14:1073267.

27   Bao Y, Zhang Y, Du C, Ji Y, Dai Y, Jiang W. Malnutrition and the Risk of Early Neurological Deterioration in Elderly Patients with Acute Ischemic Stroke. Neuropsychiatr Dis Treat. 2022:1779-87.

28.   Nam K-W, Kim CK, Yu S, Oh K, Chung J-W, Bang OY, et al. D-dimer to fibrinogen ratio predicts early neurological deterioration in ischemic stroke with atrial fibrillation. Thromb Res. 2023;229:219-24.

29   Li H, Zhang J-T, Zheng Y, Zhang D-D, Cui X-Y, Zhao X, et al. Risk factors and prognosis of early neurological deterioration in patients with posterior circulation cerebral infarction. Clin Neurol Neurosurg. 2023;228:107673.

30   Jang SH, Park H, Hong J-H, Yoo J, Lee H, Kim HA, et al. Impact of High-Intensity Statin on Early Neurologic Deterioration in Patients with Single Small Subcortical Infarction. J Clin Med. 2023;12(9):3260.

31   Shah K, Clark A, Desai SM, Jadhav AP. Causes, predictors, and timing of early neurological deterioration and symptomatic intracranial hemorrhage after administration of IV tPA. Neurocrit Care. 2022:1-7.

32.   Rodríguez-Castro E, Rodríguez-Yáñez M, Arias S, Santamaría M, López-Dequidt I, López-Loureiro I, et al. Influence of sex on stroke prognosis: a demographic, clinical, and molecular analysis. Frontiers in Neurology. 2019:388.

33   Ryu W-S, Chung J, Schellingerhout D, Jeong S-W, Kim H-R, Park JE, et al. Biological mechanism of sex difference in stroke manifestation and outcomes. Neurology. 2023;100(24):e2490-e503.

34   Girot J-B, Richard S, Gariel F, Sibon I, Labreuche J, Kyheng M, et al. Predictors of

unexplained early neurological deterioration after endovascular treatment for acute ischemic stroke. Stroke. 2020;51(10):2943-50.

35.   Kim J-M, Moon J, Ahn S-W, Shin H-W, Jung K-H, Park K-Y. The etiologies of early neurological deterioration after thrombolysis and risk factors of ischemia progression. Journal of Stroke and Cerebrovascular Diseases. 2016;25(2):383-8.

36   He Y, Yang Q, Liu H, Jiang L, Liu Q, Lian W, et al. Effect of blood pressure on early neurological deterioration of acute ischemic stroke patients with intravenous rt-PA thrombolysis may be mediated through oxidative stress induced blood-brain barrier disruption and AQP4 upregulation. Journal of Stroke and Cerebrovascular Diseases. 2020;29(8):104997.

37   Wang L, Cheng Q, Hu T, Wang N, Wei Xe, Wu T, et al. Impact of stress hyperglycemia on early neurological deterioration in acute ischemic stroke patients treated with intravenous thrombolysis. Frontiers in Neurology. 2022;13:870872.

38   Gong P, Liu Y, Gong Y, Chen G, Zhang X, Wang S, et al. The association of neutrophil to lymphocyte ratio, platelet to lymphocyte ratio, and lymphocyte to monocyte ratio with post-thrombolysis early neurological outcomes in patients with acute ischemic stroke. Journal of neuroinflammation. 2021;18(1):1-11.

39   Nam K-W, Kang MK, Jeong H-Y, Kim TJ, Lee E-J, Bae J, et al. Triglyceride-glucose index is associated with early neurological deterioration in single subcortical infarction: Early prognosis in single subcortical infarctions. International Journal of Stroke. 2021;16(8):944-52.

40   Jin D, Yang J, Zhu H, Wu Y, Liu H, Wang Q, et al. Risk factors for early neurologic deterioration in single small subcortical infarction without carrier artery stenosis: predictors at the early stage. BMC Neurol. 2023;23(1):1-9.

41   Khodair A, Fahim M, Abdelrasol I, Ahmed S. Homocysteine as a Predictor of Early Neurological Deterioration in Acute Ischemic Stroke. Benha Journal of Applied Sciences. 2022;7(11):1-7.

42.   Nam K-W, Kim CK, Yu S, Chung J-W, Bang OY, Kim G-M, et al. Elevated troponin levels are associated with early neurological worsening in ischemic stroke with atrial fibrillation. Sci Rep. 2020;10(1):12626.

43   Yu WM, Abdul-Rahim AH, Cameron AC, Kõrv J, Sevcik P, Toni D, et al. The incidence and associated factors of early neurological deterioration after thrombolysis: results from SITS registry. Stroke. 2020;51(9):2705-14.

44   Liu Y-L, Yin H-P, Qiu D-H, Qu J-F, Zhong H-H, Lu Z-H, et al. Multiple hypointense vessels on susceptibility-weighted imaging predict early neurological deterioration in acute ischaemic stroke patients with severe intracranial large artery stenosis or occlusion receiving intravenous thrombolysis. Stroke and vascular neurology. 2020:svn-2020-000343.

45   Zhang YX, Shen ZY, Jia YC, Guo X, Guo XS, Xing Y, et al. The Association of the neutrophil-to-lymphocyte ratio, platelet-to-lymphocyte ratio, lymphocyte-to-monocyte ratio and systemic inflammation response index with short-term functional outcome in patients with acute ischemic stroke. Journal of Inflammation Research. 2023:3619-30.

46.   Miyamoto N, Tanaka Y, Ueno Y, Kawamura M, Shimada Y, Tanaka R, et al. Demographic, clinical, and radiologic predictors of neurologic deterioration in patients with acute ischemic stroke. Journal of Stroke and Cerebrovascular Diseases. 2013;22(3):205-10.

47.   Amer HA, El-Jaafary SIM, Sadek HMAE-A, Fouad AM, Mohammed SS. Clinical and paraclinical predictors of early neurological deterioration and poor outcome in spontaneous intracerebral hemorrhage. The Egyptian Journal of Neurology, Psychiatry and Neurosurgery. 2023;59(1):1-11.

48   Tan C, Zhao L, Dai C, Liang Y, Liu H, Zhong Y, et al. Risk factors related to early neurological deterioration in lacunar stroke and its influence on functional outcome. International Journal of Stroke. 2023;18(6):681-8.

49   Lee H, Heo J, Lee IH, Kim YD, Nam HS. Association between blood viscosity and early

neurological deterioration in lacunar infarction. Frontiers in Neurology. 2022;13:979073.

50.   Li J, Quan K, Wang Y, Zhao X, Li Z, Pan Y, et al. Effect of stress hyperglycemia on neurological deficit and mortality in the acute ischemic stroke people with and without diabetes. Frontiers in Neurology. 2020;11:576895.

51   Kwan J, Hand P. Early neurological deterioration in acute stroke: clinical characteristics and impact on outcome. Journal of the Association of Physicians. 2006;99(9):625-33.

52.   Seo W-K, Seok H-Y, Kim JH, Park M-H, Yu S-W, Oh K, et al. C-reactive protein is a predictor of early neurologic deterioration in acute ischemic stroke. Journal of Stroke and Cerebrovascular Diseases. 2012;21(3):181-6.

53   Fang L, Wang Y, Zhang H, Jiang L, Jin X, Gu Y, et al. The neutrophil-to-lymphocyte ratio is an important indicator correlated to early neurological deterioration in single subcortical infarct patients with diabetes. Frontiers in Neurology. 2022;13:940691.

54   Ryu W-S, Schellingerhout D, Jeong S-W, Nahrendorf M, Kim D-E. Association between serum lipid profiles and early neurological deterioration in acute ischemic stroke. Journal of Stroke and Cerebrovascular Diseases. 2016;25(8):2024-30.

55   Deng Q, Li S, Zhang H, Wang H, Gu Z, Zuo L, et al. Association of serum lipids with clinical outcome in acute ischaemic stroke: A systematic review and meta-analysis. Journal of clinical neuroscience. 2019;59:236-44.

56   Choi K-H, Park M-S, Kim J-T, Chang J, Nam T-S, Choi S-M, et al. Serum triglyceride level is an important predictor of early prognosis in patients with acute ischemic stroke. Journal of the neurological sciences. 2012;319(1-2):111-6.

57   Wang Q, Jiang G, Yan L, Chen R, Liu Y, Liu L, et al. Association of atherogenic index of plasma with early neurological deterioration in patients with acute ischemic stroke. Clin Neurol Neurosurg. 2023;234:108014.

58   Arenillas JF, Rovira Á, Molina CA, Grivé E, Montaner J, Álvarez-Sabín J. Prediction of early neurological deterioration using diffusion-and perfusion-weighted imaging in hyperacute middle cerebral artery ischemic stroke. Stroke. 2002;33(9):2197-205.

59   Qureshi AI, Suarez JI, Yahia AM, Mohammad Y, Uzun G, Suri MFK, et al. Timing of neurologic deterioration in massive middle cerebral artery infarction: a multicenter review. Critical care medicine. 2003;31(1):272-7.

60   Derflinger S, Fiebach JB, Böttger S, Haberl RL, Audebert HJ. The progressive course of neurological symptoms in anterior choroidal artery infarcts. International Journal of Stroke. 2015;10(1):134-7.

61   Chausson N, Joux J, Saint-Vil M, Edimonana M, Jeannin S, Aveillan M, et al. Infarction in the anterior choroidal artery territory: clinical progression and prognosis factors. Journal of Stroke and Cerebrovascular Diseases. 2014;23(8):2012-7.

62   Donnan GA, O'malley H, Quang L, Hurley S, Bladin PF. The capsular warning syndrome: pathogenesis and clinical features. Neurology. 1993;43(5):957-.

63   Vynckier J, Maamari B, Grunder L, Goeldlin MB, Meinel TR, Kaesmacher J, et al. Early neurologic deterioration in lacunar stroke: clinical and imaging predictors and association with long-term outcome. Neurology. 2021;97(14):e1437-e46.

64   Uz A, Erbil KM, Esmer A. The origin and relations of the anterior choroidal artery: an anatomical study. Folia morphologica. 2005;64(4):269-72.

65   Nelles M, Gieseke J, Flacke S, Lachenmayer L, Schild H, Urbach H. Diffusion tensor pyramidal tractography in patients with anterior choroidal artery infarcts. American Journal of Neuroradiology. 2008;29(3):488-93.

66.   Tran AT, Huynh QH, Nguyen DM, Bui HM, Vu HD, Nguyen TV, et al. Evaluating the axonal injury and predicting the motor function recovery in supratentorial acute stroke patients. Interdisciplinary Neurosurgery. 2024;36:101919.

67.   Siegler JE, Samai A, Semmes E, Martin-Schild S. Early neurologic deterioration after

stroke depends on vascular territory and stroke etiology. Journal of Stroke. 2016;18(2):203.
68   Cui Y, Meng W-H, Chen H-S. Early neurological deterioration after intravenous thrombolysis of anterior vs posterior circulation stroke: a secondary analysis of INTRECIS. Sci Rep. 2022;12(1):3163.
69   Lee DH, Sung JH, Yi HJ, Lee MH, Song SY. Effect on Successful Recanalization of Thrombus Length in Susceptibility-weighted Imaging in Mechanical Thrombectomy with Stentretrieval. Current Neurovascular Research. 2021;18(1):78-84.
70   Grand T, Dargazanli C, Papagiannaki C, Bruggeman A, Maurer C, Gascou G, et al. Benefit of mechanical thrombectomy in acute ischemic stroke related to calcified cerebral embolus. Journal of Neuroradiology. 2022;49(4):317-23.
71.   Maurer CJ, Dobrocky T, Joachimski F, Neuberger U, Demerath T, Brehm A, et al. Endovascular thrombectomy of calcified emboli in acute ischemic stroke: a multicenter study. American Journal of Neuroradiology. 2020;41(3):464-8.
72.   Yamamoto N, Satomi J, Tada Y, Harada M, Izumi Y, Nagahiro S, et al. Two-layered susceptibility vessel sign on 3-tesla T2*-weighted imaging is a predictive biomarker of stroke subtype. Stroke. 2015;46(1):269-71.
73   Chen J, Zhang Z, Nie X, Xu Y, Liu C, Zhao X, et al. Thrombus magnetic susceptibility is associated with recanalization and clinical outcome in patients with ischemic stroke. NeuroImage: Clinical. 2022;36:103183.
74   Xuan F, Zhang M, Wenwei Y. Correlation study between early neurological deterioration and cerebral microbleeds in patients with acute small artery occlusion. Chinese Journal of Postgraduates of Medicine. 2023:488-94.
75.   Aoki J, Iguchi Y, Urabe T, Yamagami H, Todo K, Fujimoto S, et al. Microbleeds and clinical outcome in acute mild stroke patients treated with antiplatelet therapy: ADS post-hoc analysis. Journal of clinical neuroscience. 2021;89:216-22.
76.   Choi K-H, Kim J-H, Kang K-W, Kim J-T, Choi S-M, Lee S-H, et al. Impact of microbleeds on outcome following recanalization in patients with acute ischemic stroke. Stroke. 2019;50(1):127-34.
77   Berge E, Whiteley W, Audebert H, De Marchis G, Fonseca A, Padiglioni C. European Stroke Organisation (ESO) guidelines on intravenous thrombolysis for acute ischaemic stroke. Eur Stroke J. 2021; 6 (1): I-LXII. Eur Neurol. 2022;85:349-66.
78   Sousanidou A, Tsiptsios D, Christidi F, Karatzetzou S, Kokkotis C, Gkantzios A, et al. Exploring the Impact of Cerebral Microbleeds on Stroke Management. Neurology International. 2023;15(1):188-224.
79   Zhou Z, Malavera A, Yoshimura S, Delcourt C, Mair G, Salman RA-S, et al. Clinical prognosis of FLAIR hyperintense arteries in ischaemic stroke patients: a systematic review and meta-analysis. Journal of Neurology, Neurosurgery & Psychiatry. 2020;91(5):475-82.
80.   Nave AH, Kufner A, Bücke P, Siebert E, Kliesch S, Grittner U, et al. Hyperintense vessels, collateralization, and functional outcome in patients with stroke receiving endovascular treatment. Stroke. 2018;49(3):675-81.
81.   Zhu L, Gong S, Zhu X, Zhang R, Ren K, Zhu Z, et al. FLAIR vascular hyperintensity: an unfavourable marker of early neurological deterioration and short-term prognosis in acute ischemic stroke patients. Ann Palliat Med. 2020;9:3144-51.
82   Kim D-H, Lee Y-K, Cha J-K. Prominent FLAIR vascular hyperintensity is a predictor of unfavorable outcomes in non-thrombolysed ischemic stroke patients with mild symptoms and large artery occlusion. Frontiers in Neurology. 2019;10:722.
83   Lee H-j, Kim T, Koo J, Kim Y-D, Na S, Choi YH, et al. Multiple chronic lacunes predicting early neurological deterioration and long-term functional outcomes according to TOAST classification in acute ischemic stroke. Neurological Sciences. 2023;44(2):611-9.
84.   Xie X, Xiao J, Wang Y, Pan L, Ma J, Deng L, et al. Predictive model of early

neurological deterioration in patients with acute Ischemic stroke: a Retrospective Cohort Study. Journal of Stroke and Cerebrovascular Diseases. 2021;30(3):105459.

85   Lee S-J, Lee D-G. Distribution of atherosclerotic stenosis determining early neurologic deterioration in acute ischemic stroke. Plos One. 2017;12(9):e0185314.

86.   Wang C, Yi X, Zhang B, Liao D, Lin J, Chi L. Clopidogrel plus aspirin prevents early neurologic deterioration and improves 6-month outcome in patients with acute large artery atherosclerosis stroke. Clinical and Applied Thrombosis/Hemostasis. 2015;21(5):453-61.

87.   Kimura T, Tucker A, Sugimura T, Seki T, Fukuda S, Takeuchi S, et al. Ultra-early combination antiplatelet therapy with cilostazol for the prevention of branch atheromatous disease: a multicenter prospective study. Cerebrovascular Diseases Extra. 2017;6(3):84-95.

88.   Wang Y, Wang Y, Zhao X, Liu L, Wang D, Wang C, et al. Clopidogrel with aspirin in acute minor stroke or transient ischemic attack. New England Journal of Medicine. 2013;369(1):11-9.

89.   Johnston SC, Easton JD, Farrant M, Barsan W, Conwit RA, Elm JJ, et al. Clopidogrel and aspirin in acute ischemic stroke and high-risk TIA. New England Journal of Medicine. 2018;379(3):215-25.

90.   Powers WJ, Rabinstein AA, Ackerson T, Adeoye OM, Bambakidis NC, Becker K, et al. Guidelines for the early management of patients with acute ischemic stroke: 2019 update to the 2018 guidelines for the early management of acute ischemic stroke: a guideline for healthcare professionals from the American Heart Association/American Stroke Association. Stroke. 2019;50(12):e344-e418.

91   Cappellari M, Bovi P, Moretto G, Zini A, Nencini P, Sessa M, et al. The THRombolysis and statins (THRaST) study. Neurology. 2013;80(7):655-61.

92.   van Dongen MME, Aarnio K, Martinez-Majander N, Pirinen J, Sinisalo J, Lehto M, et al. Use of statins after ischemic stroke in young adults and its association with long-term outcome. Stroke. 2019;50(12):3385-92.

93   Yang W-Y, Li Y-F, Wang Z-R, Yu T-X, Xu D-J, Yang N, et al. Combined therapy of intensive statin plus intravenous rt-PA in acute ischemic stroke: the INSPIRE randomized clinical trial. Journal of neurology. 2021;268:2560-9.

94   Trial A. Randomized Controlled Trial of Early Versus Delayed Statin Therapy in Patients With Acute Ischemic Stroke. Stroke. 2017;48(11):3057-63.

95.   Yen-Chu H, Lee J-D, Weng H-H, Lin L-C, Tsai Y-H, Yang J-T. Statin and dual antiplatelet therapy for the prevention of early neurological deterioration and recurrent stroke in branch atheromatous disease: a protocol for a prospective single-arm study using a historical control for comparison. BMJ open. 2021;11(11):e054381.

96.   Siegler JE, Boehme AK, Albright KC, George AJ, Monlezun DJ, Beasley TM, et al. A proposal for the classification of etiologies of neurologic deterioration after acute ischemic stroke. Journal of Stroke and Cerebrovascular Diseases. 2013;22(8):e549-e56.

97.   Nair SB, Somarajan D, Pillai RK, Balachandran K, Sathian S. Predictors of early neurological deterioration following intravenous thrombolysis: Difference between risk factors for ischemic and hemorrhagic worsening. Annals of Indian Academy of Neurology. 2022;25(4):627.

98   Awadh M, MacDougall N, Santosh C, Teasdale E, Baird T, Muir KW. Early recurrent ischemic stroke complicating intravenous thrombolysis for stroke: incidence and association with atrial fibrillation. Stroke. 2010;41(9):1990-5.

99   Dowlati E, Sarpong K, Kamande S, Carroll AH, Murray J, Wiley A, et al. Abnormal neurological pupil index is associated with malignant cerebral edema after mechanical thrombectomy in large vessel occlusion patients. Neurological Sciences. 2021:1-10.

100.   Romagnosi F, Bernini A, Bongiovanni F, Iaquaniello C, Miroz J-P, Citerio G, et al. Neurological pupil index for the early prediction of outcome in severe acute brain injury

patients. Brain Sci. 2022;12(5):609.

101   Huang Z-X, Wang Q-Z, Dai Y-Y, Lu H-K, Liang X-Y, Hu H, et al. Early neurological deterioration in acute ischemic stroke: A propensity score analysis. Journal of the Chinese Medical Association. 2018;81(10):865-70.

102.   Simonsen CZ, Schmitz ML, Madsen MH, Mikkelsen IK, Chandra RV, Leslie-Mazwi T, et al. Early neurological deterioration after thrombolysis: clinical and imaging predictors. International Journal of Stroke. 2016;11(7):776-82.

103   Stokum JA, Gerzanich V, Simard JM. Molecular pathophysiology of cerebral edema. Journal of Cerebral Blood Flow & Metabolism. 2016;36(3):513-38.

104   Liebeskind DS, Jüttler E, Shapovalov Y, Yegin A, Landen J, Jauch EC. Cerebral edema associated with large hemispheric infarction: implications for diagnosis and treatment. Stroke. 2019;50(9):2619-25.

105   Liebeskind DS, Kim D, Starkman S, Changizi K, Ohanian AG, Jahan R, et al. Collateral failure? Late mechanical thrombectomy after failed intravenous thrombolysis. Journal of Neuroimaging. 2010;20(1):78-82.

106   Shuaib A, Butcher K, Mohammad AA, Saqqur M, Liebeskind DS. Collateral blood vessels in acute ischaemic stroke: a potential therapeutic target. The Lancet Neurology. 2011;10(10):909-21.

107.   Chen C, Parsons MW, Levi CR, Spratt NJ, Miteff F, Lin L, et al. Exploring the relationship between ischemic core volume and clinical outcomes after thrombectomy or thrombolysis. Neurology. 2019;93(3):e283-e92.

108.   Campbell BC, Christensen S, Tress BM, Churilov L, Desmond PM, Parsons MW, et al. Failure of collateral blood flow is associated with infarct growth in ischemic stroke. Journal of Cerebral Blood Flow & Metabolism. 2013;33(8):1168-72.

109   Rocha M, Jovin TG. Fast versus slow progressors of infarct growth in large vessel occlusion stroke: clinical and research implications. Stroke. 2017;48(9):2621-7.

110.   Seners P, Hurford R, Tisserand M, Turc G, Legrand L, Naggara O, et al. Is unexplained early neurological deterioration after intravenous thrombolysis associated with thrombus extension? Stroke. 2017;48(2):348-52.

111   Lemkes BA, Hermanides J, DeVries JH, Holleman F, Meijers JC, Hoekstra JB. Hyperglycemia: a prothrombotic factor? Journal of Thrombosis and Haemostasis. 2010;8(8):1663-9.

112   He L, Wang J, Wang F, Zhang L, Zhang L, Zhao W, et al. The length of susceptibility vessel sign predicts early neurological deterioration in minor acute ischemic stroke with large vessel occlusion. BMC Neurol. 2021;21(1):1-8.

113   Seners P, Delepierre J, Turc G, Henon H, Piotin M, Arquizan C, et al. Thrombus length predicts lack of post-thrombolysis early recanalization in minor stroke with large vessel occlusion. Stroke. 2019;50(3):761-4.

114   Fitzgerald S, Mereuta OM, Doyle KM, Kallmes DF, Brinjikji W. Correlation of imaging and histopathology of thrombi in acute ischemic stroke with etiology and outcome. Journal of neurosurgical sciences. 2019;63(3):292.

115   Galovic M, Ferreira-Atuesta C, Abraira L, Döhler N, Sinka L, Brigo F, et al. Seizures and epilepsy after stroke: epidemiology, biomarkers and management. Drugs & aging. 2021;38:285-99.

116   Ma S, Fan X, Zhao X, Wang K, Wang H, Yang Y. Risk factors for early-onset seizures after stroke: A systematicreview and meta-analysis of 18 observational studies. Brain and Behavior. 2021;11(6):e02142.

117   Bogousslavsky J, Martin R, Regli F, Despland P-A, Bolyn S. Persistent worsening of stroke sequelae after delayed seizures. Archives of neurology. 1992;49(4):385-8.

118   Westendorp WF, Nederkoorn PJ, Vermeij J-D, Dijkgraaf MG, de Beek Dv. Post-stroke

infection: a systematic review and meta-analysis. BMC Neurol. 2011;11(1):1-7.

119.   Xu J, Yalkun G, Wang M, Wang A, Wangqin R, Zhang X, et al. Impact of infection on the risk of recurrent stroke among patients with acute ischemic stroke. Stroke. 2020;51(8):2395-403.

120.   Suda S, Aoki J, Shimoyama T, Suzuki K, Sakamoto Y, Katano T, et al. Stroke-associated infection independently predicts 3-month poor functional outcome and mortality. Journal of neurology. 2018;265:370-5.

121   Kamel H, Iadecola C. Brain-immune interactions and ischemic stroke: clinical implications. Archives of neurology. 2012;69(5):576-81.

122   Becker KJ, Dankwa D, Lee R, Schulze J, Zierath D, Tanzi P, et al. Stroke, IL-1ra, IL1RN, infection and outcome. Neurocrit Care. 2014;21:140-6.

123   Cao Y, Wang F, Cheng Q, Jiao X, Lv X. Fasting blood glucose levels affect hospitalization time and relapse and mortality rates of cerebral infarction patients. International Journal of Clinical and Experimental Medicine. 2015;8(7):11508.

124   Lv P, Zhang L, Chen X. Pulse pressure level after acute ischemic stroke is associated with early neurological deterioration. Experimental and Therapeutic Medicine. 2024;27(2):1-6.

125   Castillo J, Leira R, García MM, Serena J, Blanco M, Dávalos A. Blood pressure decrease during the acute phase of ischemic stroke is associated with brain injury and poor stroke outcome. Stroke. 2004;35(2):520-6.

126   Ryu J-C, Bae J-H, Ha SH, Chang JY, Kang D-W, Kwon SU, et al. Blood pressure variability and early neurological deterioration according to the chronic kidney disease risk categories in minor ischemic stroke patients. Plos One. 2022;17(9):e0274180.

127   Seners P, Baron J-C. Revisiting 'progressive stroke': incidence, predictors, pathophysiology, and management of unexplained early neurological deterioration following acute ischemic stroke. Journal of neurology. 2018;265(1):216-25.

128.   Zhu Y, Wu M, Wang H, Zheng Y, Zhang S, Wang X, et al. Daily blood pressure variability in relation to neurological functional outcomes after acute ischemic stroke. Frontiers in Neurology. 2023;13:958166.

129   Jung H-J, Ryu J-C, Joon Kim B, Kang D-W, Kwon SU, Kim JS, et al. Time Window for Induced Hypertension in Acute Small Vessel Occlusive Stroke With Early Neurological Deterioration. Stroke. 2023.

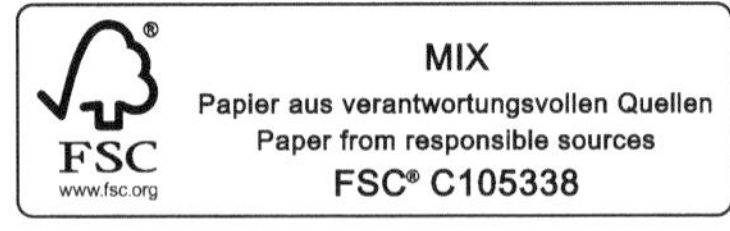

Printed by Books on Demand GmbH, Norderstedt / Germany